her sweet spot

her sweet spot

101 sexy ways
to find and please it

Jude Schell

photographs by
Janette Valentine

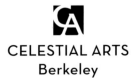

CELESTIAL ARTS
Berkeley

Library of Congress Cataloging-in-Publication Data
Schell, Jude, 1969–
  Her sweet spot : 101 sexy ways to find and please it / Jude Schell. — 1st ed.
     p. cm.
  Summary: "Equal parts erotica, bedroom how-to, and sex and relationship
miscellany, this is a guide to discovering and pleasing female sweet spots—
from the obvious to the obscure"—Provided by publisher.
  1. Sex. 2. Sexual excitement. 3. Intimacy (Psychology) I. Title.

  HQ31.S34 2010
  306.77—dc22

2010026384

ISBN 978-1-58761-006-6

Printed in Hong Kong

Design by Colleen Cain

Photography assistance by Lisa Martin-Owens
Art direction by Jude Schell
Set design by Aimée Ammon
Makeup and hair styling by Virginia Le Fay and Jessica Coury

Models: Cassandra Burton, Melba D., Ashley Garner, Jewel, Sheeba Knight,
Lisa Lehrer, Kim Linger, Aurora Natrix

10 9 8 7 6 5 4 3 2 1

First Edition

for Aimée,
who, in our seventeenth year together,
continues to give me more pleasure
(and pain)
than anyone I've ever known

CONTENTS

INTRODUCTION

Her Sweet Spot is a testament to the wonder and the beauty of women, desire, and pleasure. It's a pastiche of female sexuality at its most real and fantastic, offering a pathway to a deeper understanding of a woman's unique sensual potential.

There are so many ways for lovers to discover and enhance their capacities for pleasure. Within these pages are 101 ideas to indulge your imagination and inspire and entice you to explore. It's my hope that you find this lushly illustrated book to be a fresh, entertaining, and compelling guide that exudes her sensuality on every page.

Pleasure is derived from thoughts, actions, and experiences. Each woman enjoys various pleasures uniquely and to different degrees throughout her life. What she desires, and when and how, also constantly changes—and ideally, evolves. Even the most confident and worldly woman needs to be reminded that there's always a new pleasure to be unveiled and shared.

Sexuality and sensuality are not only ever-evolving, they're complex. Her deepest yearnings originate and lie in her mind, heart, body, and soul. Her sexual appetite, personal passions, and fundamental needs are all intrinsically linked. To find and please her countless and diverse sweet spots, stimulate the whole woman.

Her sweet spot of the moment may be her clitoris, her love of romantic settings, or her preference for a sexual encounter featuring light bondage—it will range from the obvious to the elusive. Her sweet spot is a blend of her physical, sexual, emotional, psychological, and spiritual natures. Finding and pleasing one sweet spot often leads to the arousal of another. To find her sweetest spots, the places on and within her that long to be *touched*, every aspect of her nature must be explored in the most sensorial way. As you uncover her proclivities and reveal her desires, going on to attend to and fulfill them all is also a dynamic enterprise—and sweet fun.

Making sense of the senses through a better understanding of her unique nature increases her capacity to know the most and best sexual pleasure. To inspire her to develop her sensual abilities and strive for heightened awareness, *Her Sweet Spot* investigates her attitudes, instincts, dreams, and her body and its responses to all she sees, smells, hears, tastes, touches, and feels.

Falling in love is easy. Staying is love is hard. Pleasure is a priority, like good health, purpose, fulfilling relationships, and meaningful connections. Value her sexuality, and respect, acknowledge, and embrace its complicated nature, and the rewards will never stop flowing.

Deep bonds between women occur on every level. Across the globe, women are giving and accepting pleasure, and confidently reshaping their world around their desires. Women are growing more perceptive, powerful, expressive, and satisfied every day. *Her Sweet Spot* is designed to create a sexy, funny, and smart atmosphere to stimulate a woman's motivation to pursue, experience, and enjoy—at minimum—101 paths to pleasure.

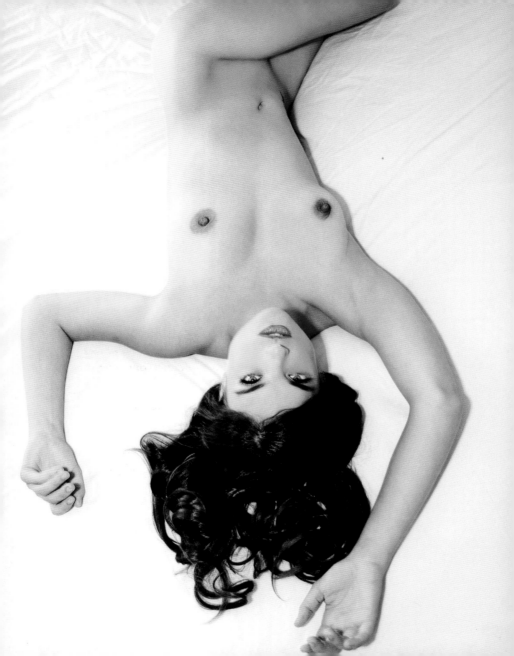

1 Stop and Smell the Flower

Keep the channel open.

She desires what pleases her senses.

She pursues what she imagines will fulfill her urges.

Passion stems from desire, and many waking hours are spent seeking to satisfy the yearnings that desire stirs.

Live sensorially.

Be aware of the subtle aspects of the world around you.

A faint yet powerful scent causes you to pause, inhale deeply, and endeavor to identify its source. An infectious laugh at a nearby table grabs your attention. You turn and catch her eye, and a connection is made.

Impressions are formed within seconds, yet can last a lifetime.

A single choice has the power to transform everything going forward, for both you and her. Any second can be *that* second—when everything you know as real is turned upside down. And it's wonderful!

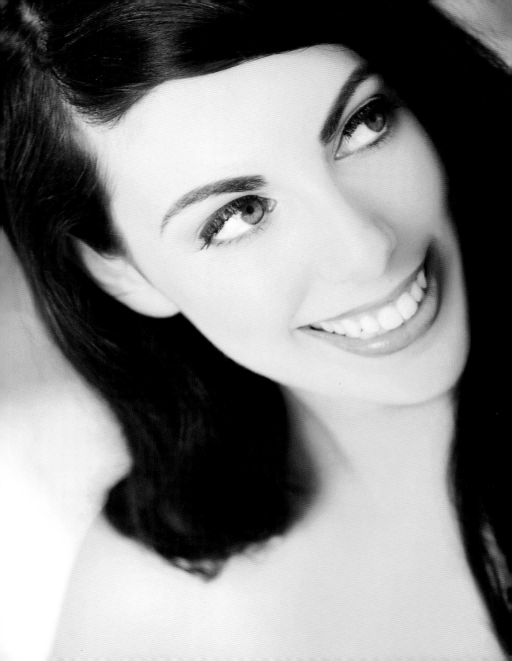

② Pitching the Woo

Love shouldn't be left to fate.

Flirting is fleeting. Charm is transformative and everlasting.

She longs to be and feel successful, interesting, and desired. She's susceptible to doubts and *shoulda woulda couldas.*

Engaging her in conversation affirms her ability to attract. And your efforts to entertain and enthrall her convey ambition—and the confidence to pursue what you want.

A sincere compliment acknowledges strengths and counters apprehensions. In this comfortable state of mind she's open to continuing flirtatiousness, and can go on to envision an assortment of pleasing scenarios that will unfold between the two of you.

Charm is one part innate, one part studied and honed.

To captivate her mind, body, and soul, mix up the woo, interspersing insights with enticing innuendos and enchanting turns of phrase.

Be direct.

I've noticed you around, and find you very attractive.

Be playful.

Did you invite all these people?
I thought it was going to be just the two of us!

Seduce the mind to seduce the whole woman.

3 Wit

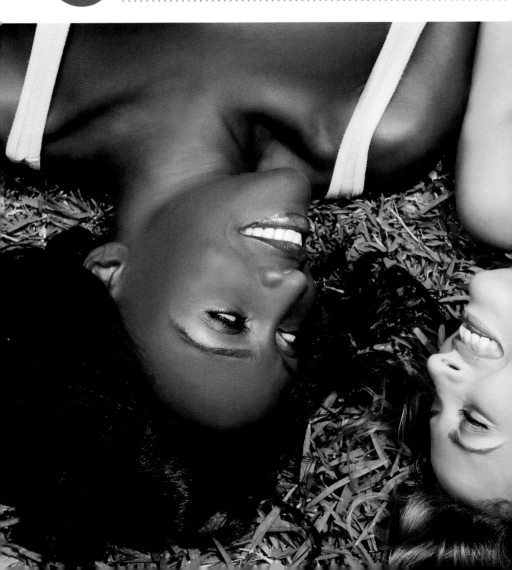

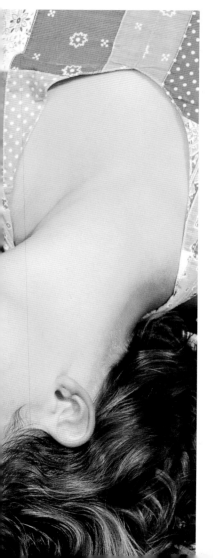

Make her laugh, genuinely and out loud.

Laughing releases serotonins, the feel-good-all-over neurotransmitters that alleviate stress and promote better sleep, memory, and mood.

Serve it up **dry and nutty, fruity and fresh.** Dedicate time to improve your ability to discover nuances and make intelligent connections between ideas. Introduce cleverness with ease.

Express your plucky view of the world concisely. As Shakespeare reminds us, *Brevity is the soul of wit.*

Even the wittiest are not always quick on their feet. Keep a couple of quips, quotes, lines of snappy dialogue, and **anecdotes in your pocket.** Be inspired by the wit and wisdom of Dorothy Parker, Oscar Wilde, Winston Churchill, and Mae West.

A tickling of her funny bone dissolves inhibitions and clears the way to tickle much more.

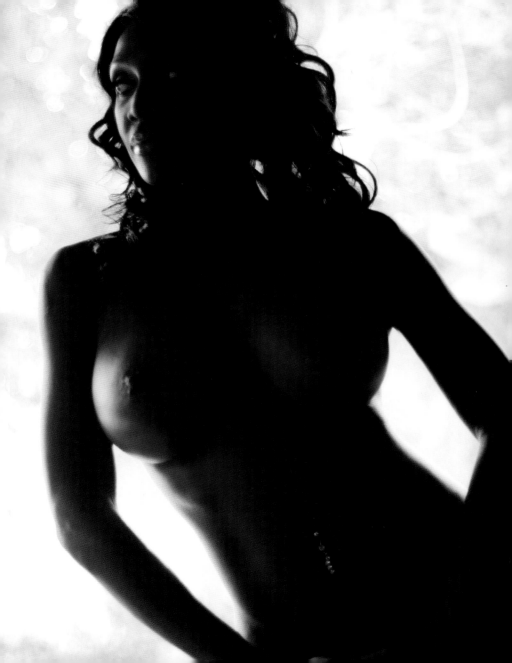

4 Glow

Physical attraction almost always happens first, but what shines forth from within you determines your staying power.

We're instantly drawn to those whom others want to be around. **Become the woman whom other women want to know, want to be, and want to be with.**

Your body is a pleasure instrument designed to receive and transmit a wide range of sensory stimuli. Activate your sensorial equipment, both genetic and neural, through sexual self-actualization. Once you recognize and embrace pleasure, you can go on to direct and control the positive energy you emit and absorb.

She'll lose her heart in the lavender haze, instantly and forever, to the rare and alluring woman who radiates beauty, sensuality, and eroticism.

5 **The Eyes Have It**

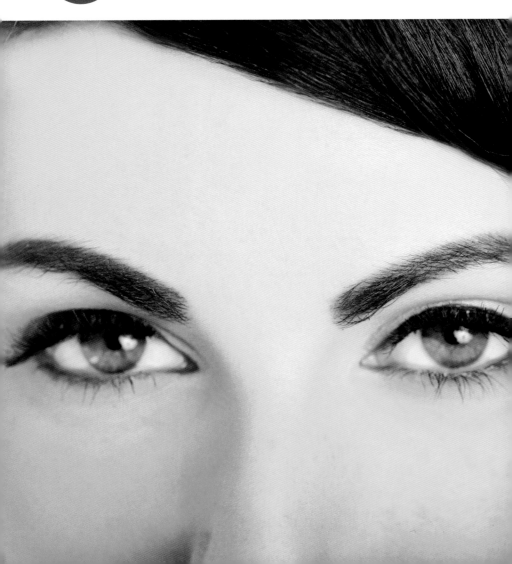

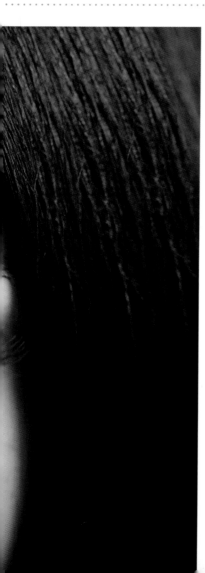

Intelligence, influence, attitude, intent . . . your **eyes reveal your center.**

You're attracted to her. A glance and then a steady gaze leaves little room for misinterpretation, especially if she's the one to look away first.

Smile. A smile truly does light up a room.

Lock eyes to gain her trust and respect.

Once you've caught her eye, maintain the eye contact while attending to something else, such as unhurriedly pulling on a pair of gloves, or tying or removing your scarf.

Wink at her.

A bold wink is always exciting. It conveys that the two of you now share a secret. It's a hint of something more.

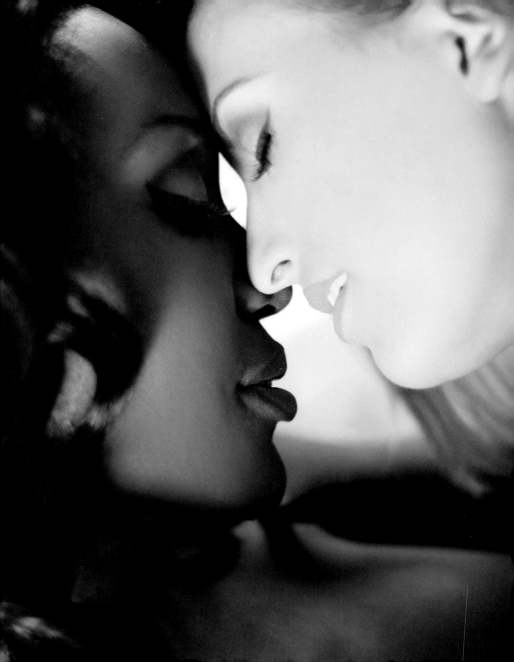

6 Kiss Kiss Bang Bang

Kisses fulfill an array of intentions. Lips press against another as a greeting or farewell, to seal a pact, for good luck, and to express respect, fondness, attraction, passion, and love.

Kissing is a vital element in the chemistry of love. **A woman's decision to take another woman as her lover** relies greatly on the sensations she experiences when their lips first meet.

You've both been imagining the first electric instant when your racing minds and lust-filled bodies fluently merge, mingle, and meld. Relax, and let this irreversible, sink-or-swoon moment unfold naturally. **What's natural is nearly always what's most extraordinary.**

As you and she continue to smooch, your lips will increase in sensitivity. And when the mutual pleasure grows into combustible arousal, your lips will swell.

The way you kiss should always be a very special thing to her.

7 Temptress

Stoke her desire to know you by craftily planting **the seed of intrigue.**

Make an impression and then disappear into thin air—bait, nibble, and no fish!

Fawn and then be gone.

Be a challenge. Remain an **elusive, unattainable vixen** for as long as is possible and practical.

Dominate her thoughts as she contemplates the mystery of you, enumerating your compelling qualities again and again in her mind.

Feeling on the other side of the world, she impatiently wonders where you are, what you're doing, and when she'll be with you again.

She fantasizes that you, her object of desire, are lying next to her, and imagines the many **irresistible, sensual pleasures that lie in wait** for you both when at long last, you reemerge for her to claim as hers.

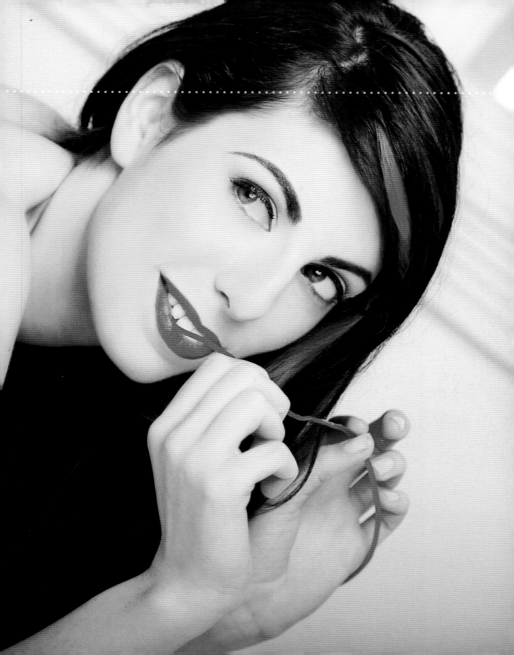

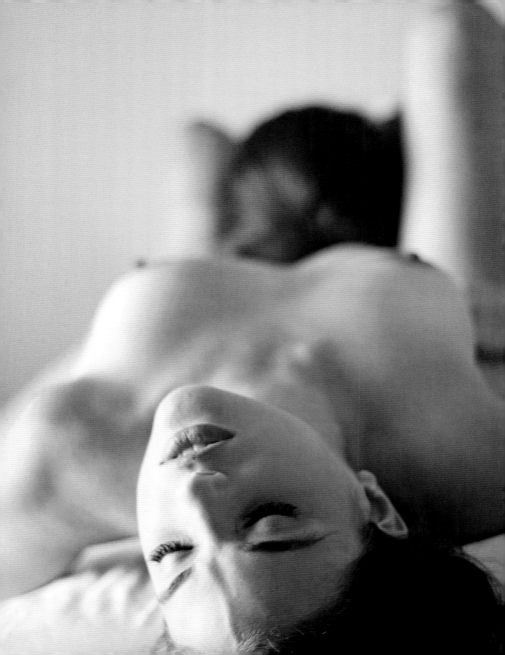

8 Ripple Effect

No two orgasms will be exactly the same.

Orgasmic energy often travels as it's released, sending shudders throughout her body. A woman's orgasm usually lasts about twenty seconds, yet after an intense sensual connection, her **afterglow** of dynamic sensations can pleasantly pulsate for hours.

She's capable of *status orgasmus*, a sustained or expanded orgasm. In 1966, William Masters and Virginia Johnson detailed a woman's forty-three-second orgasm, consisting of an estimated twenty-five successive contractions.

The brain can only store so many of the neurotransmitters released during a climax, therefore it's unusual for her to have a prolonged orgasm of more than a minute—but she might.

It's agreed that her ability to climax will increase with age, yet researchers haven't reached a consensus on the types and sources of the female orgasm. Tune in to her sensorially, and vary the atmosphere, sex position *du jour*, props, toys, and techniques to offer her the greatest opportunities to experience **climax after extraordinary climax.**

And always, send her to slumber with love and affection; she may orgasm while she sleeps, and as she dreams.

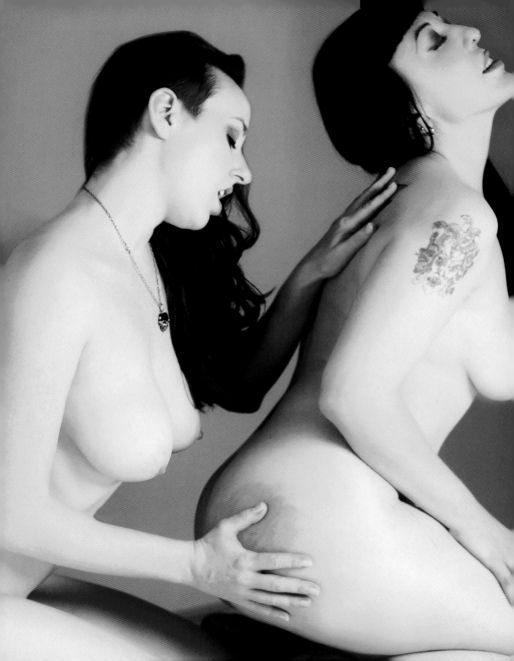

9 Spank

Your cheeky lover deserves your pronounced blows for being so **super-spankaliciously seductive.**

Spanking, generally considered light BDSM, can be a provocative vignette or the encounter's main event.

BDSM is an acronym encompassing bondage and discipline, dominance and submission, and masochism. These inclinations can be acted out in countless scenarios with varying degrees of seriousness and intensity.

Emotion, pain, behavior, memory, and the senses are all processed in the brain's limbic system. Thus her body, facilitated by her nervous system, responds to pain and pleasure in much the same way. Your spanks will flood her brain with euphoric endorphins, speed up her blood flow, stimulate her libido, and enhance her pleasure.

Run your nails across her blushing *derrière*, aiming for the area away from the anus, and then give your sweetheart another loving swat to inflame her already keen nerve endings.

The sexiest sound of the **perfect palm-to-fanny union** can be achieved by holding your hand loosely and cupping it just right.

Alternately, use a paddle or hairbrush to propel the shock waves of invigorating **jouissance** way beyond her enticing twin cheeks.

Stimulus combinations produce original and exhilarating sensations. **Cup her pussy** with your free hand, or position a toy or prop to press against her enthusiastic clitoris each time you give her bottom another reverential *thwack!*

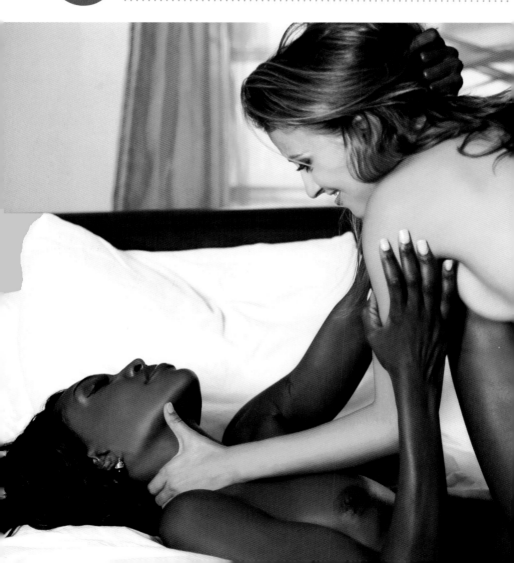

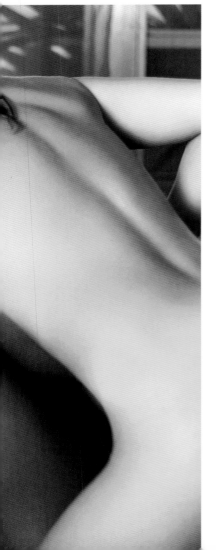

Take it slowly and let it build.

Make her as restless as a greyhound in the slips, bringing her to the brink until she's so primed to bolt out the gate and release herself into waves of orgasmic pleasure that it's virtually unbearable.

Deliberately delay her gratification.

As you taste her luscious muff, understand her responses—her heat, her wetness, the tensing of her body, and the swelling of her breasts and pussy. When her legs tighten around your head as she nears a climax, lighten the pressure of your tongue and begin to gently explore her outer labia.

As **she tingles with anticipation,** yearning to know the bliss that's so near, teasingly say,

Relax!

Thwart her efforts to raise her hips and press her insistent pussy into your warm mouth before returning to her full, wet flower. Bestow upon her **the fulfillment she aches for—complete release.**

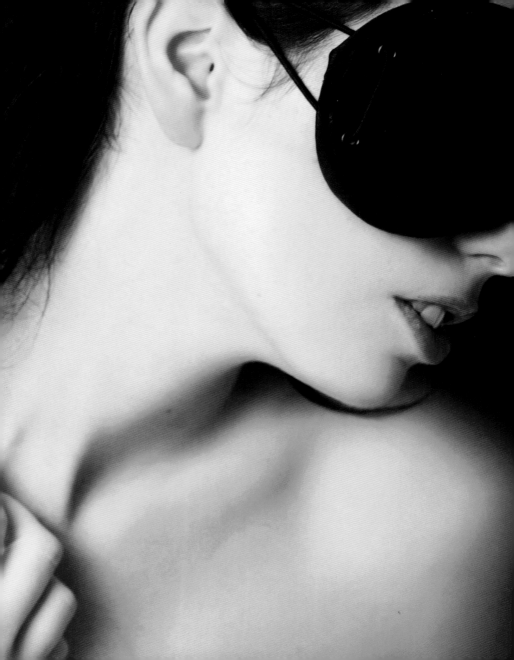

11 Deprive

Sensory deprivation incites her imagination and fuels her love of intrigue.

What's she planning to do to me?
Where will she touch me next?

Take it slowly and move smoothly, as surprises are delightful but startling can be alarming. Whisper provocatively into her ear as you drizzle massage oil onto her back and your front, sexing up the bare surfaces that are about to meet.

Her other senses will compensate for her suppressed sense of sight. **She'll breathe you in** as you playfully bite her shoulder and then run your tongue along her neck to her earlobe. She'll anticipate the warmth of your skin long before you press your body against hers.

Kiss her deeply as you caress her breasts and run your hands down her body and along the curves of her hips. Move your lips to her nipples.

A woman experiencing sensory deprivation tends to open up and become suggestible. Use this opportunity to **explore unusual erogenous areas,** such as the crease behind each knee, her wrists, her armpits, and the small of the back.

Take her hand, guide her fingers to your soft, wet *lower lips,* and whisper,

Feel me.

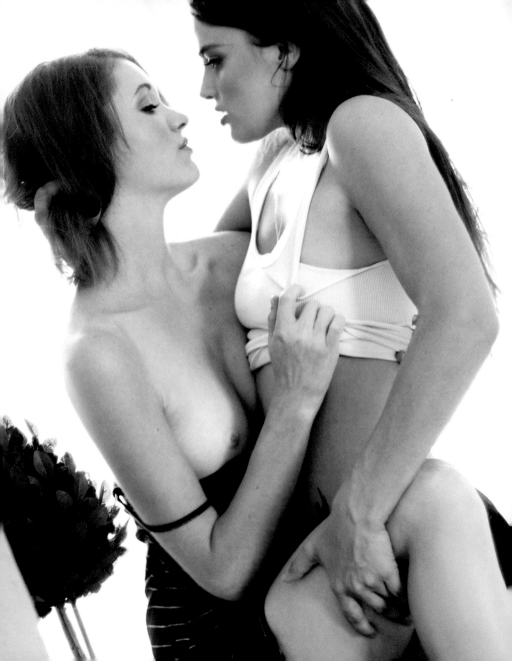

12 Sexual Body Language

Listen to her body.

As her sexual pleasure grows, her . . .

. . . breathing elevates.

. . . heart rate increases.

. . . temperature rises.

. . . muscles tense.

. . . breasts grow in size, including her areola. Nipples harden.

. . . labia minora expand and darken in color; labia majora flatten.

. . . vagina lubricates itself as its walls become smoother. It also expands, although when nearing climax, her opening narrows.

. . . clitoral glans becomes swollen, protrudes from its hood, and then withdraws slightly as her excitement plateaus.

Focus. As you fuck her with your fingers or toy of choice, does she grip you tightly? Meet your thrusts? If the answer's yes, you're either **doing it just right** or **she wants it harder.**

To enhance her own pleasure and yours, she can perform a *pompoir*, **flexing and squeezing** her supple vaginal muscles around your fingers. Those who move too fast miss this remarkable opportunity to receive **the most intimate of all hugs.**

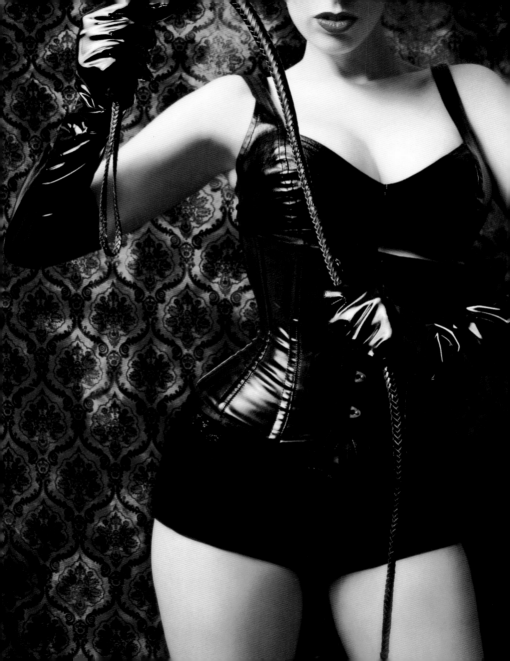

13 Tell

No one can truly know what goes on in another woman's mind.

The **power of the pussy** is daunting. Fearing she'll disappoint, she could choose to risk less—and avoid talking openly about how to bring the pussy the most and best pleasure. **It takes a real woman to ask for directions.**

The appetites and experiences of lovers will never be identical and are always changing. **Individual desires can become shared desires** only when lovers freely communicate.

An excellent way to encourage her to voice her most intimate wishes is to tell her what *you* want—and when and how.

Language is powerful. Tell her to do that certain thing she does so well—that sexy move with her hands, body, or mouth that never fails to send you over the top. Tell her how she makes you feel.

Remember that time . . . and what you did to me . . .

Tell her when it's good. Plead for more.

The more certain she is that she's pleasing you, the more she'll want to. And the more she'll grant you every splendid opportunity to discover all the wonderful ways you can satisfy her.

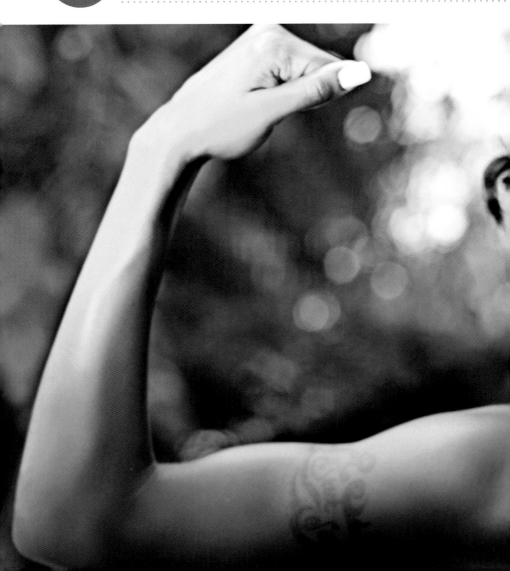

Do It . . .

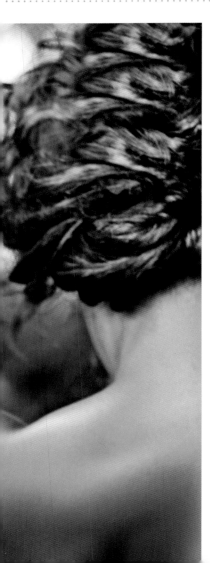

The actions of individuals **propel history.**

According to legend, eleventh-century temptress and arts advocate Lady Godiva shed her inhibitions for change. Her nobleman husband agreed to ease the people's crushing tax burden on the condition that she demonstrate what he felt to be her frivolous conviction—that **art can raise consciousness.**

Inspired by the ancient belief that a nude body is one of the highest expressions of nature, she shamelessly rode bare through the marketplace, forever transforming the perceptions of her spellbound audience.

Heroes fill us with purpose through their examples. **Inspiring people inspire.**

Mahatma Gandhi urged us to *be the change you want to see in the world.*

Exhibit the courage to act according to your principles. The more she hears about and sees your actions of merit, the more she'll want to know, and want to do, both alone and with you.

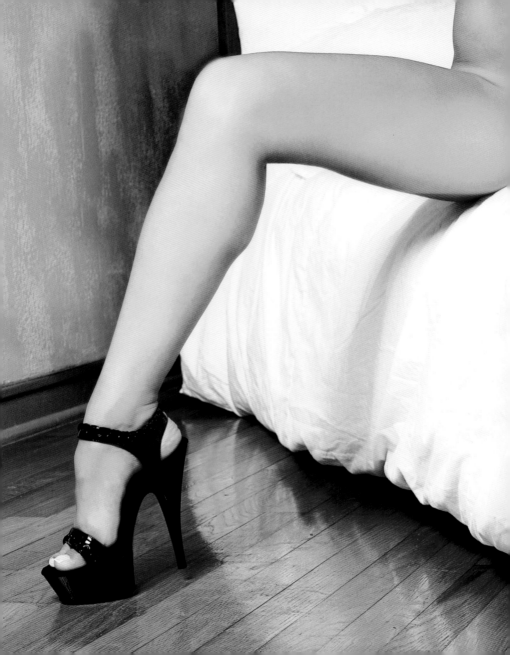

15 Show

A woman is responsible for her own sexuality. The ability to **delight, thrill, and fulfill** both herself and her lover is intimately tied to an awareness of her own body, needs, and longings. *Jilling* or *jillin' off* is a woman's essential technique for stirring and satisfying her own sweet spots.

Women climax most frequently from jilling.

Offer her a voyeuristic buzz. Invite her to a private performance and show her how you master your own domain.

As you stimulate and pleasure yourself, take her hand, slide it between your open legs, and press her fingers against your clit and into the folds of your vagina. Allow her to explore and excite you, saturating her fingers with your wetness. **Feel her feel your heat,** each response, shudder, and shiver as your arousal grows, and—ultimately—the throbbing of your post-orgasmic pussy.

Even the most enlightened and experienced partner will benefit from a *hands-on* course. Swap roles and ask her to guide you in the particulars of her sensual happiness.

Touch it. Taste it. Breathe it.

Live it to know it.

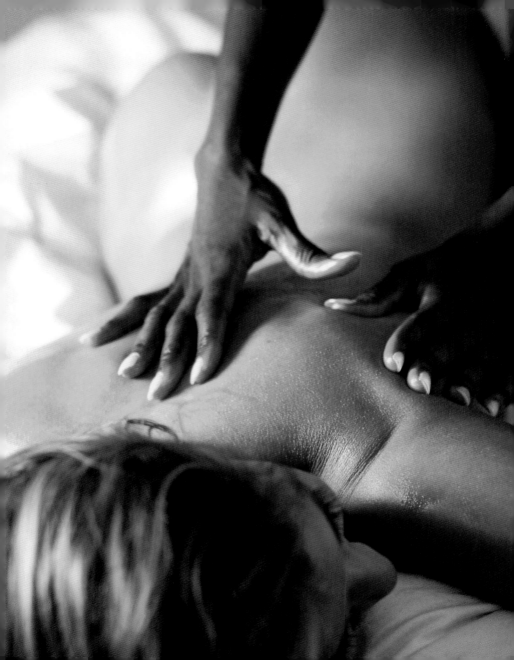

16 Sublimate

The influence of the brain on all matters sexual is indisputable, yet many declare skin to be the largest sex organ. **Pay homage to her delicate epidermis** through body sublimation.

In her daily maneuverings, she likely relies the most on her sense of sight. However, to initiate, explore, and enjoy sex and sexuality, she swears by her sense of touch.

Purposeful touch releases tension in her body and her mind, clearing the way for her sensual nature to emerge. **Luxurious skin-to-skin** contact also moves her energy, improving her circulation and overall wellness, both of which are intrinsically tied to sexual performance and satisfaction.

Ayurveda identifies more than one hundred *marmas* (vital points just beneath the skin), which connect the mind and body. Nearly a third of these *marmas* are in her head and neck area. Lavish time and attention on this region. You can release her sensually paralyzing emotional stress with a well-executed neck nibble.

As **she surrenders to the sweetness of tranquility,** your skillful hands transporting her to a place of euphoric exaltation, gift her the inevitable *happy ending.*

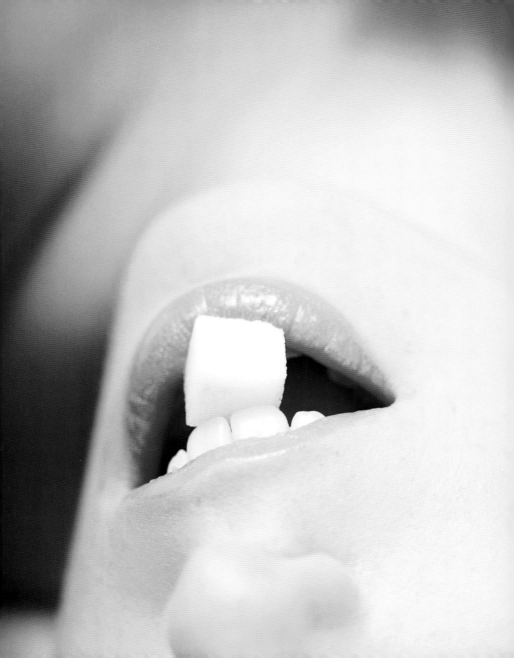

17 Sugarcoat

Overload her pleasure center with **a light dose of sensory inundation.** Receiving simultaneous messages from different parts of her body will intensify her ecstasy.

Pop a sugar cube into her mouth, flooding her taste buds with **sweet, sweet pleasure.**

Drizzle fragrant massage oil along her naked body and slowly, evenly spread it over her.

As she sucks on her slowly dissolving treat, slide down to orally pleasure her. After a nice bit of licking, offer her another cube.

Reach for a vibrator, turn it on low, and press it onto her clitoris. As the vibrator hums, slip your lubricated fingers inside her vagina and passionately move them in and out of her canal, caressing its walls.

Circle her nipples with your moist, warm tongue.

When you harmoniously **pique all her amplified senses,** fantasies in her mind vivify, the aromas of oil and sex become more acute, and your moans and sighs of desire vibrate distinctly in her ears.

It's a soft explosion of **candy-coated euphoria.**

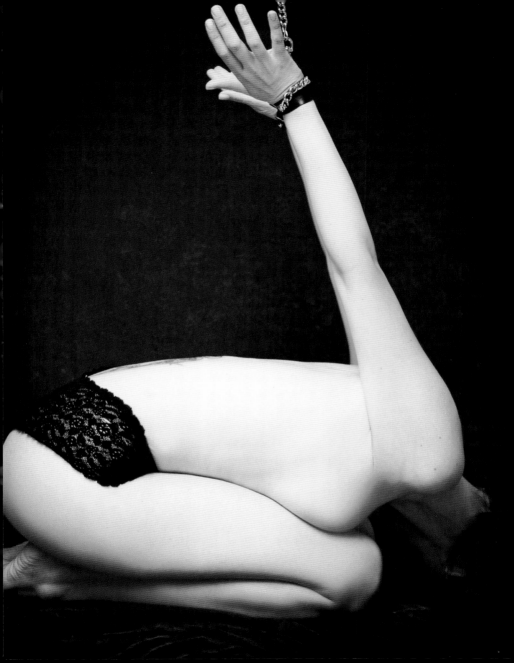

18 Awaken a Latent Desire

Unlock her clandestine door to an electrifying world.

Women may believe that they know quite well who they are and what they want, yet most aren't aware of at least some of their proclivities and desires.

Self-discovery is ongoing as **proclivities evolve.** What turned her on in her twenties may well not do it for her in her forties. What she wanted on Friday she may not be into on Tuesday.

She wasn't told,

> *You're going to transform yourself into a magnificent woman who loves to have her pussy licked while she's blindfolded and bound.*

She must continue to discover and create herself.

Her body can feel an array of sensations that her mind will interpret in a multitude of extraordinary ways. Prevent her desires from staying hidden and her sensory abilities from remaining uncultivated.

Lead her to dare to **uncover, discover, and unleash** her ever-evolving sensual potential—**to know and be more.**

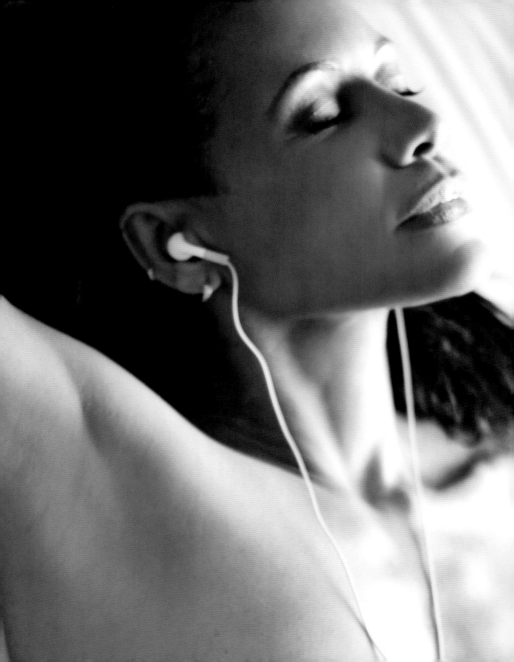

19 Music to Her Ears

The communicative and connective powers of music are so deeply felt that they transcend global boundaries and even time. Music evokes and conveys emotions that need no translation—regardless if these feelings are personally familiar, or, as of yet, unknown.

Ask her about her musical journey—what she remembers listening to as a child, the songs she enjoyed throughout her youth, and what she prefers now. Then surprise her with a music mix that transports her back to when she was perpetually carefree.

Plug in together and walk through the city while listening to the same tunes. Whether an ambient composition or energetic staccatos, this shared soundtrack will inspire **rhapsodic revelations** about your everyday surroundings.

Later at home as you fuck to the beat, sing her praises, expressing how much you totally groove on her *crescendo*.

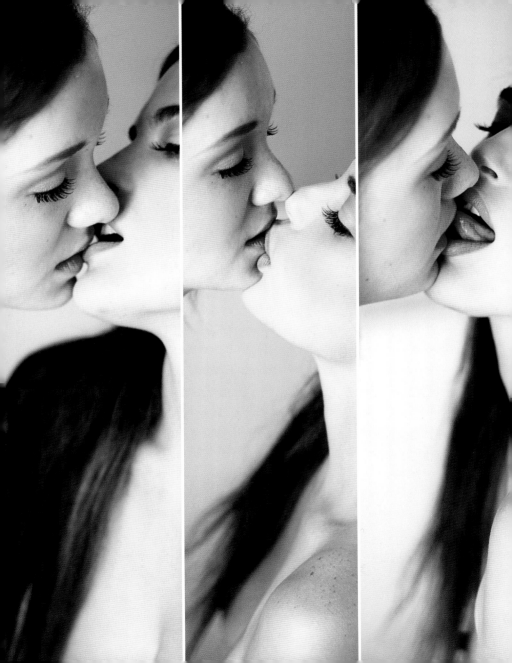

20 Demonstrate on Her Lips What You Want to Do to Her Pussy

We were saying good night. Kinda making out. Suddenly she started circling my mouth with her tongue. Then she bit down and pulled on my bottom lip with her teeth, looked me in the eyes, and smiled. I was surprised. I smiled back. She's so excellent. Really sexy. Then she slipped her tongue inside my mouth and we kissed hard. There was this kind of—I don't know—urgency. Demand. Then she closed her mouth and slid her lips back and forth across mine. Wow. It was so fuckin' hot. Then she plunged her tongue back inside my mouth, and we were kissing hard again.

I was so turned on.

Suddenly I just knew that she was pretending she was going down on me. She was licking and tonguing my pussy! Not my mouth.

I remember feeling myself start to flex my pussy muscles. Funny. I think it was some sort of half-hearted attempt to get control of myself.

We started out saying good night, and all of a sudden we were in the middle of this game. Out of nowhere. We were both throbbing.

I slid my hand into her pants and cupped and caressed her pussy through her panties. It really made me want her lips and her tongue on my swelling clit.

Brush her hair with an assured yet soothing rhythm. This loving act is sensual in and of itself.

Wet her hair and then gently squeeze out any excess water. Pour the shampoo, perhaps infused with an exotic fruit or other invigorating aroma, into your palm before applying.

Make her purr with a combination of vigorous and sensuous rubbing and circular motions. Occasionally inquire softly,

How does that feel?

Lightly run your nails across her sensitive scalp, which will usually be extremely receptive to such stimulation.

Rinse. Then comb and methodically massage conditioner through her hair.

I love your hair. It's so soft and healthy.

Rinse her hair again. Wrap her in a fresh towel.

Though this intimate encounter is about indulgence and release, when sharing something so personal, she may also become exceptionally sexually charged.

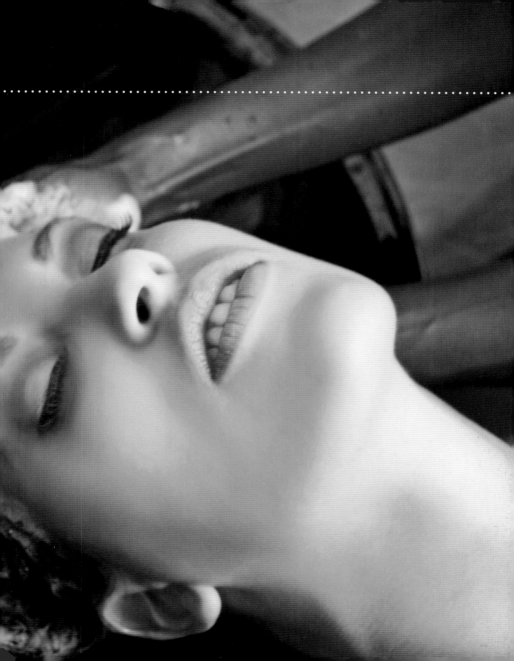

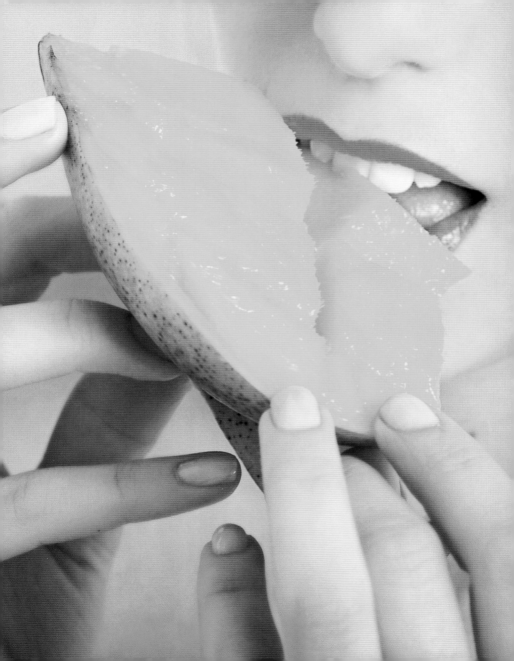

22 Epicurious

A woman of taste rarely consumes for mere sustenance. She knows that genuine gratification is derived from an abundance of excellence.

And excellence results only when each and every essential component comes together to create a mouthwatering whole.

After the loving, cook for her. The pathway to her heart is intrinsically linked to her stomach. Abundantly stimulate all her appetites and satiate her every hunger.

The sweeping experience of **sex will heighten all her senses,** most notably enhancing her sense of smell and hypersensitizing her taste buds. She'll be primed for and **craving more deliciousness** as you proceed to **please her palate** with an explosion of complex flavors, provocative aromas, and surprising textures.

The fig, a voluptuous ambrosia evocative of nectar, has long been revered for its sensual qualities. Serve your sweetie a delectable dish of thinly sliced fresh fig adorned with equally thin slices of creamy chèvre, warm or chilled.

Sex and food are two of life's most celebrated pleasures.

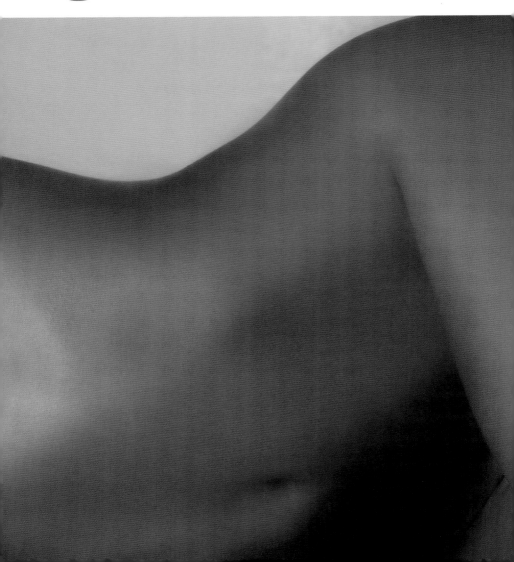

The hip is a particularly sensual area for tapping into and celebrating her energy.

Curvaceous **hips are unique to women** and grow fuller as she matures. Prominent female hips have been emphasized for thousands of years, everywhere from classical art to contemporary fashion.

Crouch before her, holding her firmly by the hips, your thumbs pressing into her. **You want her. Let her feel your hunger.**

Pull her toward you and **suckle her curves.**

As she lies on her side, admire her hips. **Run your hand along her topography.**

As she lies back on a pillow that raises her to that ideal angle where her *hoo-ha* aligns perfectly with your mouth, embrace her eminent hips for **a leisurely session of delicious pussy pleasure.**

24 Lips

The full, glistening lips of a woman's mouth can evoke fantasies of the full, glistening labia that encircle her vagina. Every woman enjoys a unique pair of these petal-like folds, the labia majora and the smaller minora within the majora, both of which serve to protect. Her minora also swell when she's aroused, enabling a tighter grip on your inserted fingers or a sex toy.

Lustrous lips resemble an open door, prompting a natural urge to enter. Her invitation to do so conveys acceptance, approval, and attraction.

The shade of lipstick or gloss that a woman wears at any given time hints prominently at her nature. The suffragists wore red lipstick as a symbol of their newfound influence. Marlene Dietrich combined a striking lip color with a traditionally masculine wardrobe and an androgynous hairstyle—contradictory elements that magnified her astonishing seductive power.

Feature your lips with an understanding of their ability to display alternate personas and express unspoken messages. When watching you speak, smile, or pucker, she'll find herself drawn to you, even if consciously she's oblivious of your *lower lala*.

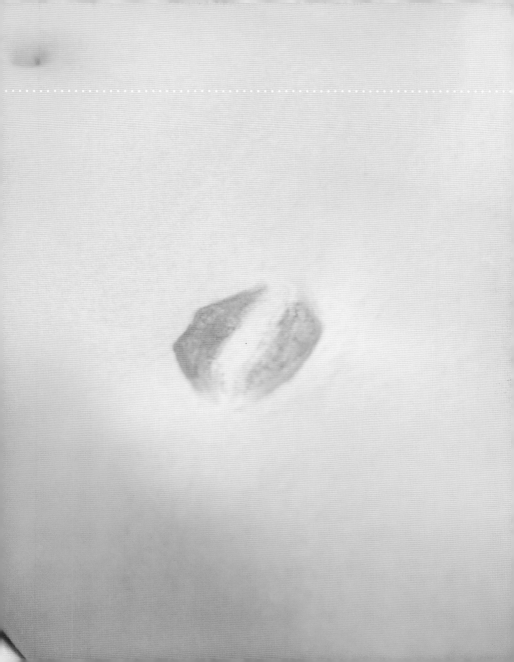

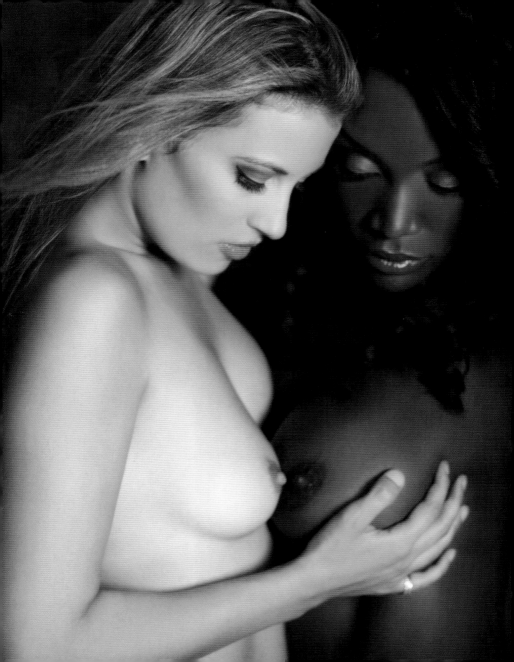

25 Tits

Some women climax from breast play alone. Others can take it or leave it.

Fondle, flatter, caress, cup, and kiss her breasts and cleavage—gently at first—lovingly exploring the expanse of this revered territory.

Move your lips and tongue around her areolae before targeting the nipples with a delicate nibble.

Women with smaller breasts often claim amplified sensations, likely due to the more concentrated nerve endings prominent on the underside of their breasts and around the nipple and areola. Thus, the bigger her breasts, the more you can anticipate a need to assertively handle *her girls* for her ultimate pleasure.

Sensitivity in a woman's breasts intensifies if her nipples are pierced, during a menstrual cycle, as she becomes sexually aroused, and after she orgasms.

Don't limit breast play to foreplay. Revisit throughout the sexual escapade. Her erect, **insistent nipples defy you** to resist an encore round of tonguing her titties.

Love those *tatas*.

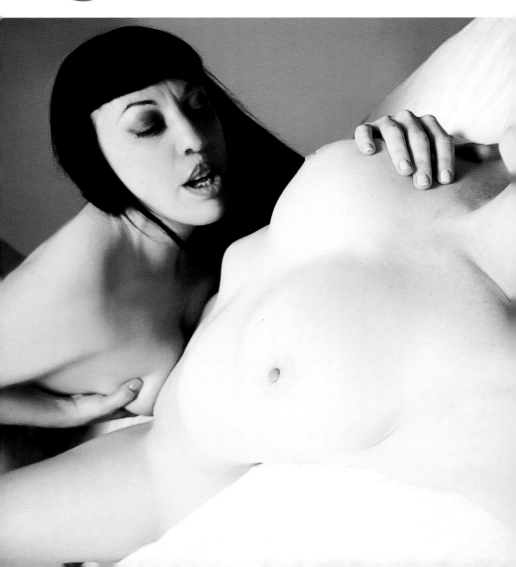

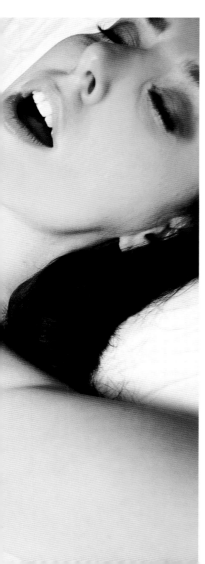

Nipples, with their fine follicles and concentrated nerve endings, are **designed for sensory delight.**

With the palm of your hand, brush across the tips of her lovely breasts. **Even slight contact has an impact.** Depending on the length of your hair, sweeping your soft locks across her chest is also exciting.

Cup your own breast in your hand and press your nipple into her *lower lady love*. Totally turn her on by pinching your nipple between your fingers to more effectively **direct it to her energized clitoris.**

Boost this sexy *nip tuck* technique with *tribadism*, simultaneously rubbing your vulva up and down her leg, adding to the shiny trail of your arousal with each pass.

Dip into **her natural emission of passion** with your fingertip, and use her own juices to glisten her nipple.

Then, **lick it off.**

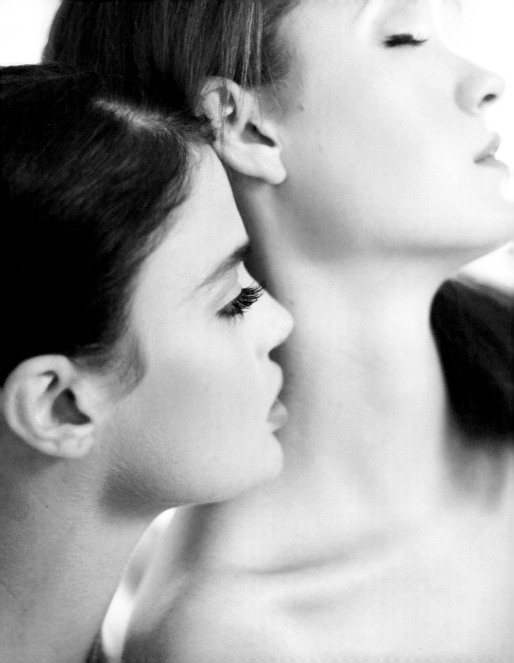

27 The Lure of Her Neck

Our culture has long exhibited a fascination with the vampire. It's exhilarating to imagine being bitten and feasted upon to thrill and sustain this exotic, impassioned creature.

The neck is a primal area for expression. **Sexual arousal from biting** is called odaxelagnia.

When she invites you to bare your teeth and indulge in this vital area of her body, she trusts that you're going for her jugular with the sole intent of subduing her with endearment. She knows that this is a reckless exposure to danger, yet she chooses it. This bewildering decision—coupled with the startling sensation that races through her body when you bite her defenseless skin—produces in her a powerful surge of passion.

Alternate light bites with licks and nibbles. Never pierce her precious skin, and adhere her signal if it becomes extreme. Take care to leave no trace, only a passing redness as **a lingering indication of your gnawing desire.**

For your finale, deliberately bite down, just beneath her shoulder—a move that will literally **give her goose bumps.**

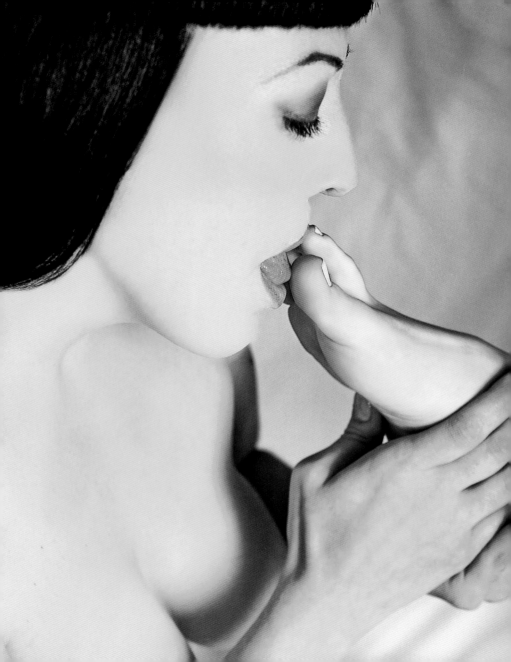

28 Knock Her Off Her Feet

The female foot has tremendous sexual power.

In 1992, *The Daily Mirror* gleefully published photos of the Duchess of York, topless and having her toes sucked. A scandal ensued, and the British royals and much of the public loudly proclaimed a distaste for this natural, rather unassuming act.

Everyone sucks for nourishment, comfort, and pleasure.

Oral sex plays a principal role in most women's sexual gratification. Skilfully sucking her toes isn't as essential as your mouth's ability to please her pussy, but the act is nearly as personal.

Run your tongue in between her toes. Treat each of her protruding toes as a phallus, **an embodiment of nature's generative power,** not unlike fingers and the clitoris.

Toe-play frequently leads to sex.

As she lies on her back with her legs raised, turn it up a notch. Continue to **tongue her toes while you greet and enter her** enthusiastic *little duchess.*

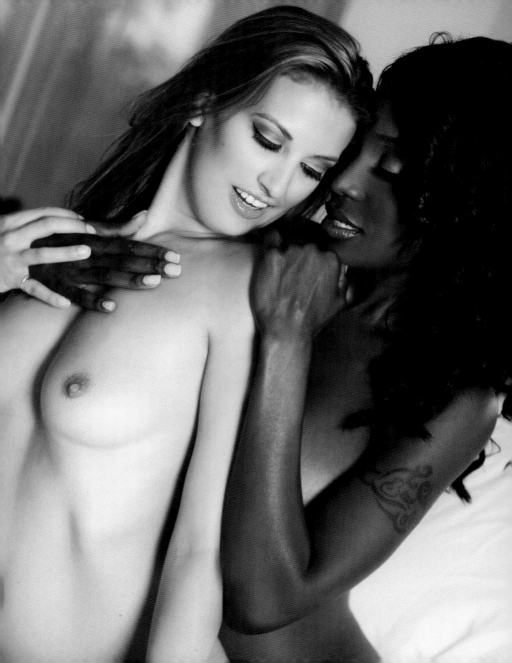

29 Talk the Talk

She may decide within the first moments of hearing you talk whether you could be her appropriate match. The voice is a rather incisive indicator of origin, status, personality, and frame of mind.

A woman favors an even voice and one that's similar to her own. Unconsciously, this preference addresses a "like seeks like" desire for harmony and self-affirmation. She'll more readily pursue connections with a woman of similar background who shares her values.

Sound commands a response. **Aurally evoke** provocative imagery. Elucidate what you're thinking, so that she can explicitly envision your fantasies and desires.

> *This rain reminds me of you. How you taste. I want to lick your fresh dew off your perfect flower.*

A **sexy play-by-play** of your arousal arouses her. Guide her in pleasuring you with a whisper. Tell her how **lovely and amazing** she's making you feel.

Whether your voice is breathy, tender, or throaty, she'll react to it with deliciously **sumptuous bedroom purrs.**

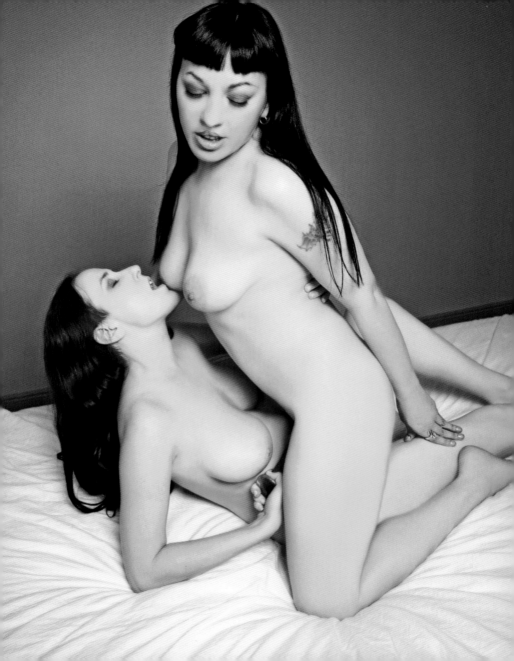

30 The Feeling Is Mutual

With mutual *jillin'*, lovers give each other a hand or finger themselves, simultaneously narrating the progress of their individual pleasure trips toward the magical queendom of Climactica.

Reach your zenith together while orally pleasing her by fiercely rubbing your clit up, down, and around on her leg and against her pelvic bone.

> *I'm gonna come. Are you ready?*
> *Tell me when you want to come.*

Engage in a *double header* and share an orgasm by simultaneously orally pleasing your *little papayas* until you come in each other's mouth—a potent dose of **mind-bending sensorial sexiness.**

To climax in harmony, you may need to modify your pace of arousal. Incorporate vibrators into the sport when one paramour is on the brink and the other's heating up gradually.

She'll quickly catch up when direct pressure is applied to her fussy pussy.

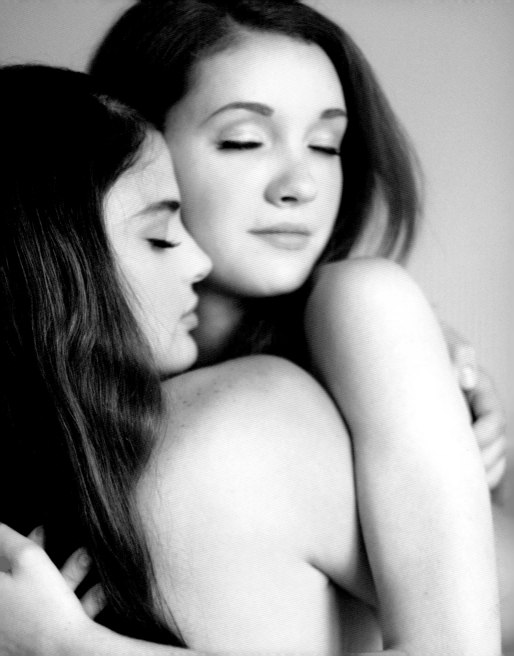

31 Treasure the Pleasure

Beauty is what you love. And **beauty in women is endless.**

A woman will attach strongly to those who continually nurture what she perceives to be her best self.

For your relationship to flourish, meet her needs again and again. Celebrate her every day—even established bonds need reinforcement.

Openly admire her; appreciate her strengths and successes. Remind her of the value she adds to the world.

Her desire is complex, ever-changing, and as recent studies affirm, not particularly tied to her physical arousal. Sparking her sometimes elusive desire is much more a matter of properly stimulating her mind.

Your warm greeting, stress-releasing caresses amid repartee, and a well-placed kiss and nibbling of her *biscuit buns* is just the catalyst she needs to awaken her overwrought senses and, to her pleasant surprise, incite her hankering.

She may forget what you say or do; **she'll always remember how you make her feel.**

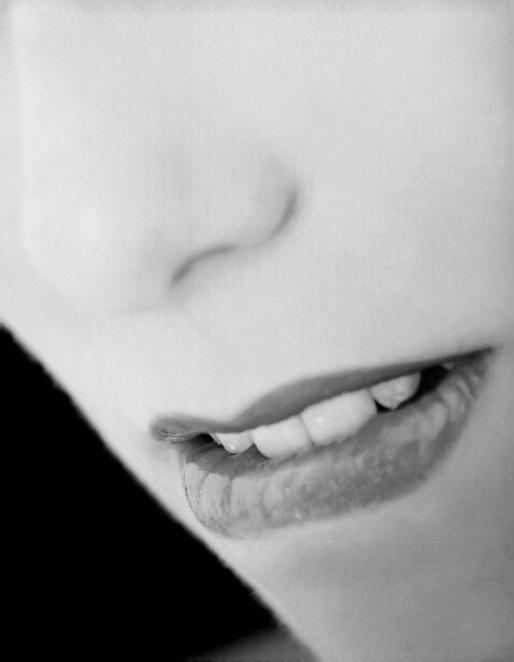

32 Heaven Scent

Scents seduce. Cleopatra flaunted her authority by dosing the fabric foils of her barge with fragrance to manipulate all that inhaled her presence as she regally floated by.

What a woman smells will dictate her mood and how she'll remember an encounter, be it trivial or significant. **Her sense of smell is primary in creating her world and is profoundly linked to her sexuality.**

Pheromones, emitted to signal and influence attraction, may powerfully penetrate her subconscious—yet these unreliable measures of sexual chemistry and compatibility are beyond your control. **Pursue the infiltration of her very essence** by nosing into the time-honored clout of the snout.

Her response to even a subtle whiff of a scent, whether strong and light or fresh and floral, and on your body or in the atmosphere, will forever be unpredictable and susceptible to innumerable influences. Experiment with mood-altering and aphrodisiacal essential oils and aromatics to enhance and transform your encounters.

Lavender is a universally-acknowledged turn-on. A hint of almond or coconut reassures her by wafting an exotic yet warmly familiar aroma. Rosemary is a stimulant, and grapefruit and pear induce happiness.

Apply your signature fragrance to attract her to favorite, erotically inclined places on your body. A dab of lush, mature sandalwood oil blended with joyful jasmine, the use of which dates back thousands of years, emits a feisty scent known to jump-start a lackluster libido.

I like the way you smell. I love the way you leave your scent on me.

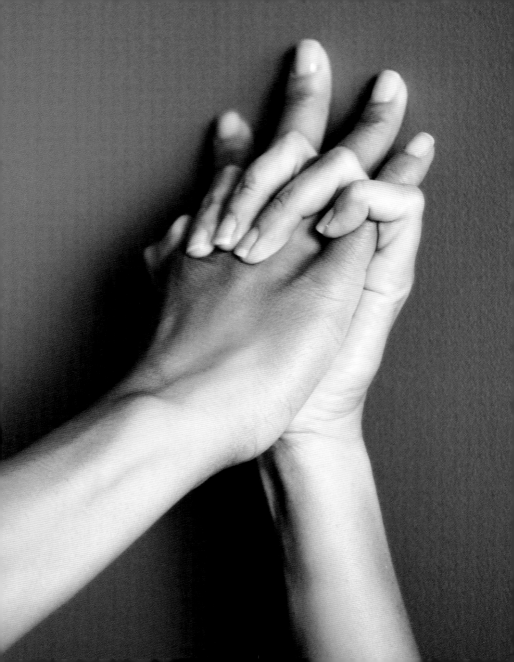

33 Effleurage

Women notice other women's hands.

Fingertips are highly sensitive to texture, moisture, temperature, pressure, and movement. Also extremely flexible, fingers are arguably a woman's most versatile sex accessory.

Treat her to an impromptu hand massage. You can give her this innocuous pleasure virtually anywhere—at home, at the movies, or in the car while waiting in a drive-through queue. Lotion or oil is preferred, but not required.

Begin with *effleurage—***a delicate yet assured caressing of her hand.** Use small, circular motions, moving along the length of each finger toward its sensitive tip. Gently squeeze and then pull each one just as you release it. Press and hold your thumb into her palm.

Beyond the obvious virtues of relaxation, wellness, and connecting, your attentive touch may incite her to imagine these same smooth, strong fingers strumming her more secluded sweet spots.

Many a woman swears that, **hands down,** nothing gets her off to a flying start and then accomplishes the mission like **a lover's adept fingers.**

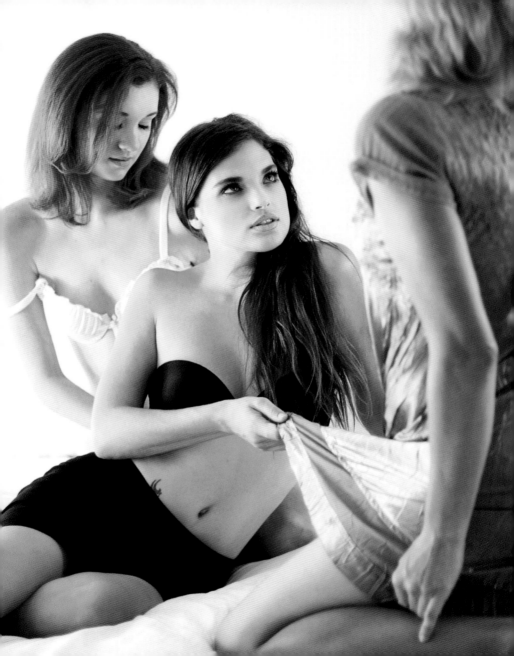

34 Threefold

Three pussies, six pairs of lips, thirty fingers, and twenty-four thousand clitoral nerve endings! Mmm . . .

A multiple-partner sexual encounter is **a notorious erotic fantasy.**

Monogamy isn't monotony, but intimacy doesn't require seclusion. There are many options in the pursuit and sustaining of great sex.

Some believe that the energy in a shared *game of flats* has more erotic charge than a twosome ever could. Yet caveat emptor, as the dynamics of polyamorous groupings are far from simple. Emotions can run high, and expectations fall short as often as they're met.

To select your third party voyeur or participant, you might invite a friend with whom both of you feel an affinity, answer an ad, or go cruising together. Even if the hook-up is impromptu, take a preliminary moment together to review the risks and rewards of a love triangle to establish sexual etiquette and boundaries.

Sexual adventurousness is enticing, and an occasional *treble play* will spice up the everyday. Take it off the glass shelf and try it on—it could just be the perfect fit.

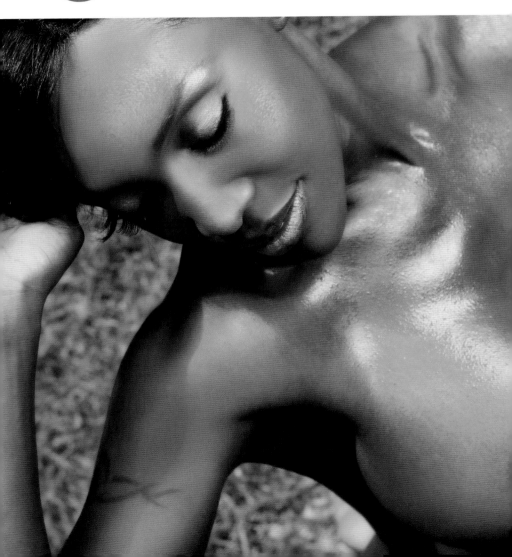

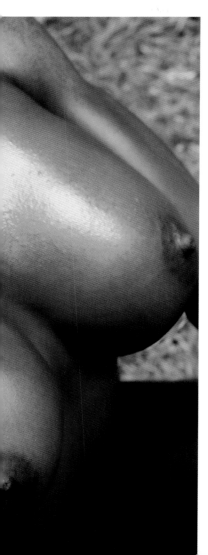

Get amped. Forget the romantic bubble bath. Go for an aphrodisiacal jog.

After a workout, lovers are revved up and revitalized. While you're still buzzing from a brisk walk on the beach or supercharged kickboxing class, bask in each other's healthy glow.

Sweat tastes both salty and sweet. Run your tongue along her chest, slipping it into the sexy ravine between her breasts.

Cup her buff buttocks with both hands, and pull her close. Initiate a round of carnal calisthenics.

See and feel her **shimmering back muscles ripple** as you grind on her taut quads. Admire the dimples in the crooks of her cut arms as she flips over and tops you, playfully pinning you down, a sheen highlighting her alluring skin.

Feel her **droplets drip down** onto you.

Thrusts, lunges, push-ups, squats, and curls take on inspired new meanings when performed between the sheets.

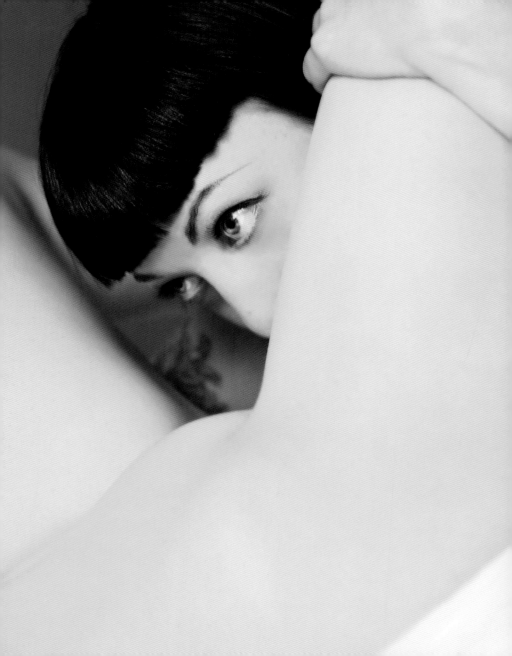

36 Whet

It's been said that the sexual appetite of the goddess Venus was first whet when her lover went down on her.

Giving good mouth involves much more than bringing her to climax. Show her that you're hard-wired to please her pussy. You know your way around. Before diving for her pearl, explore nearby. Squeeze her labia between your lips. Taste her inner thighs.

Using your fingers, spread her labia to lift her clit to your lips. Your versatile tongue is an ideal texture for sex. Flit, flick, press, release, and then hold it against her pleasure center. Tell her how much you enjoy **savoring her sweet sugar** as your tongue enters and maneuvers inside her. Then, slip a finger or two, or three, inside and continue the in-and-out rhythm. Stroke her vaginal walls with your fingertips as you return your mouth to circle the head of her clitoris. Slip your tongue under its hood.

When the rhythm's working, sustain it. Match the momentum with the pace of her arousal. When you're unsure, ask.

Once she's **on the verge,** use deliberate tongue strokes, again and again, focusing pressure on the emerging tip of her clit, which boasts more than eight thousand nerve endings, more than any other part of her body. **It exists solely to give her pleasure.**

I love eating your pussy. I've been thinking about this all day.
I want you to come in my mouth.

Lick her into shape to make Venus hum.

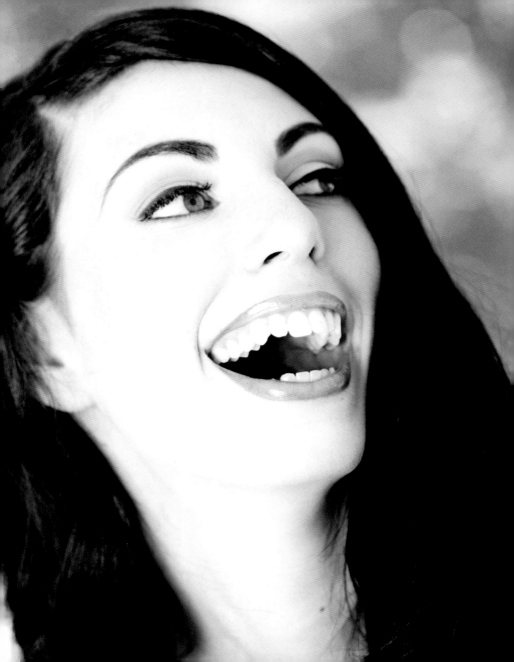

37 Tilt Her Paradigm

Within predictability lies comfort and ennui. Do the unanticipated. A jolt out of the clear blue sky overcomes the lull of her day. And unusual connections form an enduring, enthralling impression of you, the conveyor of surprise.

Effortless spontaneity is sexy. Once you arouse her curiosity she'll want to know what makes you tick. She'll wonder why and how you decide to do what you do.

Anything new causes her brain to release dopamine, a molecule that's both a stimulating neurotransmitter and a hormone. This forerunner of adrenaline and close companion to the brain's pleasure and reward system lets loose when she listens to the latest music, takes the scenic route, is given an unexpected gift, or embarks on a sexual expedition.

Take her around the bend with a shocker that'll tilt her sensual world. Slip a couple of fingers between her *labiacious petals* while *sipping her rose.* As her journey progresses, fill her *cookie jar* with your ladyfingers. With your other hand, circle and stimulate the edges of her anus with a lubricated finger, and say,

Tell me when you want to come. I know you're close. I can taste and feel that—I love that. Then I'm gonna slip my finger in just before you climax. Just a little ways in. Let's see how this makes you feel.

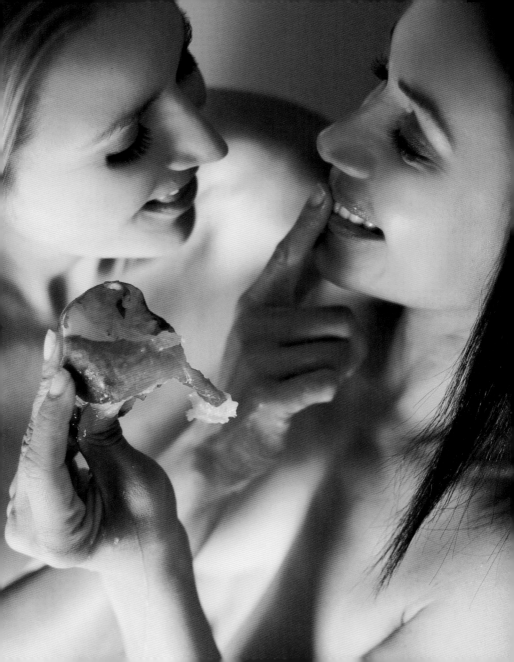

38 Slurpee Peaches

Induce her sexual hunger with a **lavish, orgyesque banquet** worthy of ancient Greece or Rome.

Serve her peaches, pomegranates, dates, apricots, cherries, berries, and pears, as well as slices of mouthwatering citrus fruits, such as grapefruits and clementines.

Lay out this spread as elaborately or modestly as you prefer—**the decadence is in the occasion.** Choose as accompaniments breads, nuts, olives, cheeses, and wine or sparkling water.

While reclining (this feast is to be enjoyed on silk cushions, not sitting at a rigid table), play games in keeping with the amorous atmosphere. Compete in **a saucy bout** of naughty-word Scrabble.

Salacious talk blends nicely with all this titillating tastiness. Riff about the sensorial experience; describe how her sugary kiss is transformed as she slurps and sucks on each particular pleasure. Write an ode to a **sticky, warm, or tart treat.**

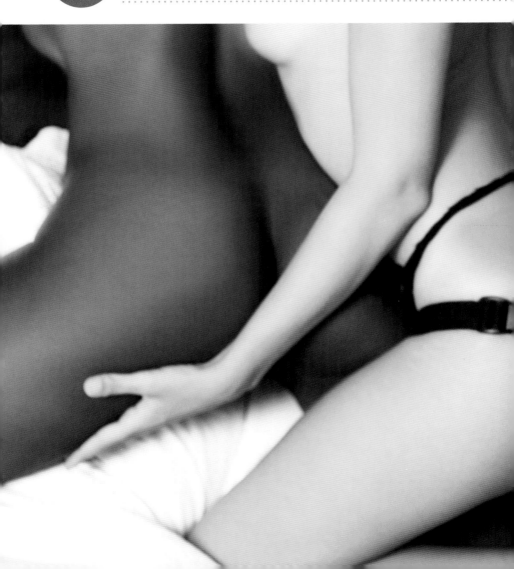

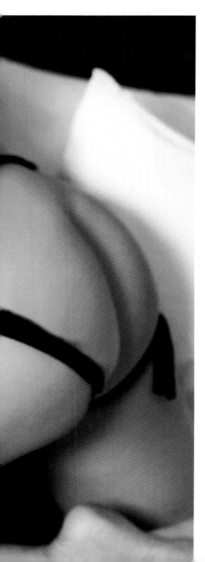

A bond is created when lovers share **the thrill of a traditionally taboo act.**

Even when not entering her, a significant degree of trust must exist to allow you to stimulate and explore her delicate, highly erogenous *tail zone*.

Leisurely slide a well-lubricated dildo **up and down between her luscious cheeks.** Tease and excite the multitude of desirous nerve endings in and around her ass.

Sexy **derrière dalliances** loosen her up physically and mentally, giving her plenty of time to anticipate forthcoming penetration, if that's indeed what the lovers agree to try as **their next forbidden feat.**

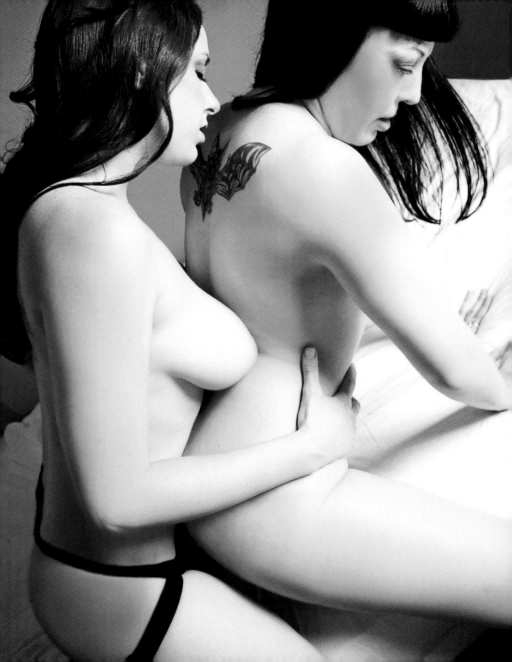

40 Knocking on Her Clit's Back Door

Sure, her clitoris exists solely to provide her pleasure; however, **this powerful lotus stem of love isn't the only game in Blisstown.**

Diversify to introduce new sensations. Devote a day to finding and pleasing *her clitoris's back door*, also known as the urethral sponge or G-spot.

Its unique texture can be felt through her vaginal wall, about a third of the way up behind her pubic bone. Curl your inserted fingers slightly toward her belly button to press up and into this concentration of erectile tissue, glands, and ducts that envelop her urethra.

Her *pleasure sponge* will swell with fluids and become firm and prominent as she's aroused by your unyielding strokes.

The size, sensitivity, and ideal angle for ultimate satisfaction vary among women. **Experiment.** Numerous toys are ergonomically designed to stimulate this region. She may also find that **when she's on top,** while you lie on your back and **fuck her upward,** she can best control the precision of penetration.

Enter her from behind, standing, kneeling, or lying on your sides, for a perfect angle to guide your *strap-on clit extension* or handheld sex toy to her target. And as the wall between the anus and vagina is thin, anal sex can also awaken her *magic spot* with a roar.

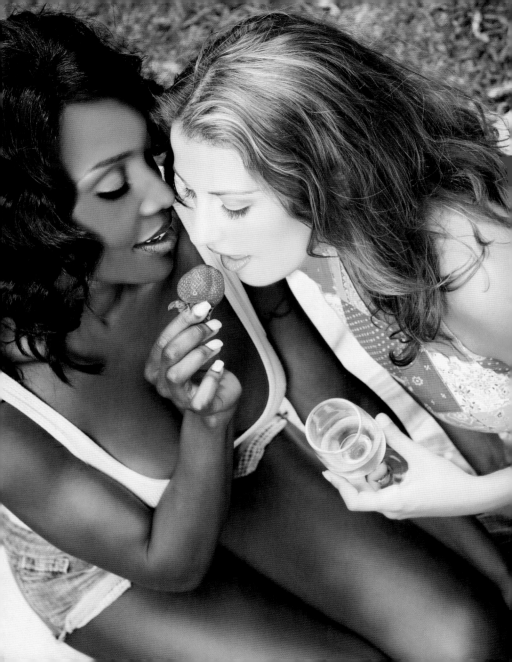

41 Where the Bee Sucks, There Suck I

What better way to tap into your sensual dispositions than to have **a three-way with Mother Nature?**

Immerse yourselves in the idyllic, seductive offerings of the great outdoors. A fresh breeze, leafy trees, blue water, a field of lavender, chirping cicadas, and an urban rooftop all provide superb ambience for lusty lovers.

Interact harmoniously with the living, breathing energy that surrounds you. Touch and be touched. **Epiphanies arise from the minutiae of life.**

As her eyes glisten with an enthusiastic sense of wonder, steal a kiss during a warm summer rain. Whisper *love* at the skies.

Pitch a tent in the magnificent redwoods, or stargaze in your own backyard. Hike toward romance with a view and fool around at a high altitude. Get busy on each other as you float in a boat.

Dip into her *honey pot* while sprawled on a bench in a private and fragrant jasmine garden.

Affirm for her that *the grass will always be the greenest here, with you.*

Frolic with her where the forecast is always **sunny with a likelihood of sizzle.**

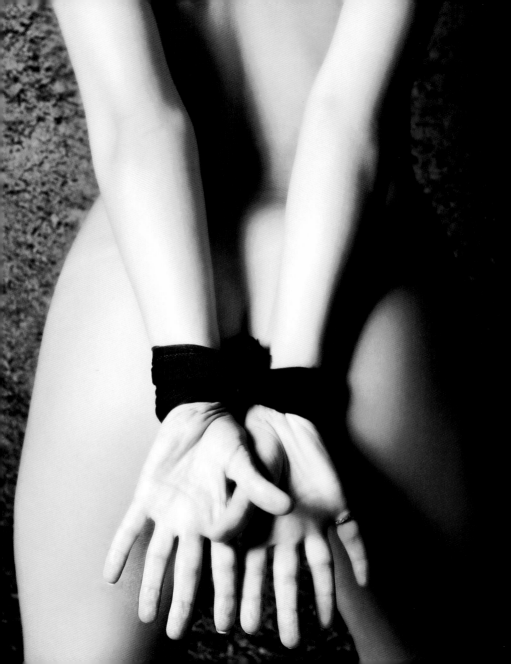

42 Touche Pas

Expose a temptation, but keep it just out of reach. **Tension is a key element in the art of seduction.**

Deny her ability to act—her ability to touch. Bind her wrists, perhaps to the bed, with silken stockings or scarves.

Play with yourself as she watches. Tease with all your favorite pleasure points.

I'm getting so wet.

Run your moistened finger down her chest, circling a nipple. Then touch yourself again and put your finger into your own mouth.

Press your pussy against her body and slide it up and down. When she battles temptation, she'll only want it more. Her attempts to resist or curb her enthusiasm will prove futile. **Her desire will transform itself into a need.**

Through tantalization, lovers maintain a mutual fascination and keep expectation alive.

Leave her something to wish for—ideally, more of something she knows and likes. Continue to deny her the ability to touch you, but let her taste your wetness. Then pull away and bring yourself to climax, either on her or as she watches, while **the taste of you lingers on her lips and in her mind.**

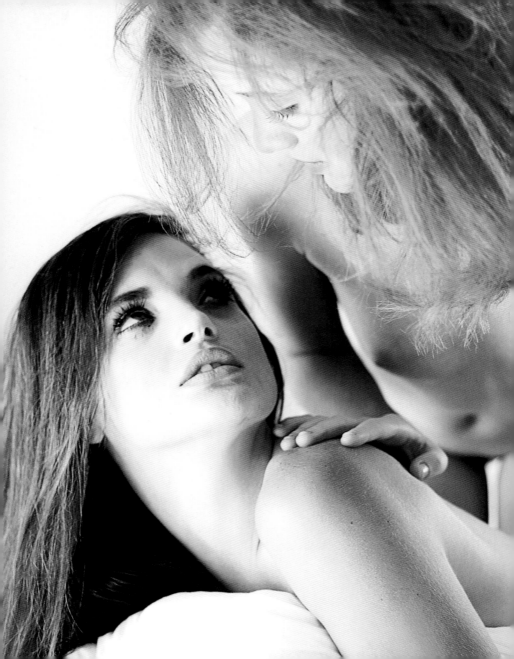

43 Fight, Flight, or Fuck

In the words of the fierce and politically progressive humanitarian Eleanor Roosevelt, *do one thing every day that scares you.*

Passion arouses her biologically and psychologically, so she immediately feels a need to *fight, flight, or fuck.*

Shock, love, confrontation, and fear all create passion. This enduring emotion is one of the most compelling and intense that a woman can feel. Passion explains, for example, her attraction to a dangerous person, as well as her inclination to mistakenly associate her ensuing arousal with sexual desire, infatuation, or even love. **Danger, like pleasure, exhilarates.**

With a lover, *fight, flight, or fuck* is just that. Her body is primed for any of these. She'll ultimately choose, consciously or not, whether to fight, flight, or fuck as the momentum of her feel-good, confidence-boosting endorphins and heart-racing, lust-inducing adrenaline surge through her.

Danger opens her up to *forbidden* emotions. **A flash of daring transports her** to that instant when she's living purely in the moment—an ultimate state of aliveness. Thus she'll always seek a thrill, all the while fundamentally desiring a life of security.

Ride a roller coaster for **a taste of danger followed by a release and return to safety.** The fleeting fear converts into sexy passion as your mutual screams morph into glee. Accelerate her experience by fingering her *naughty bits* during the wild ride, mixing the energy of the mechanics with the turbulent forces of passion.

A relationship that's as exhilarating as it is reassuring is forever.

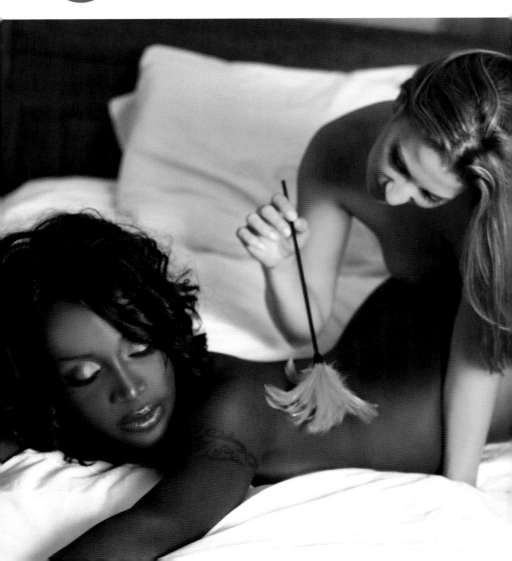

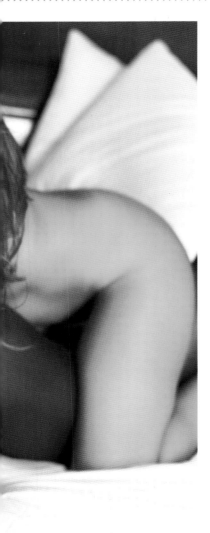

Sensuality is powerful and fragile.

Get her derailed sensuality back on track and **bring every inch of her body to attention** in the most tender way—with sensory play.

Props boost sexual thoughtfulness and vivify the drama of any sexy situation. Awaken her usual and unusual places with a feather, an artist's paintbrush, or a blush brush.

Build trust as she consents to a full exploration of her luscious body. Delicately brush her face and neck. Sweep her sensitive forearm and tickle her armpits, tummy, and inner thighs. Discover how her ears, nipples, anus, the tops of her feet, and the tips of her toes respond to your subtle touches, teasing jabs, and hypnotic circles.

Take your sweet time so she can relax, savor each moment, and express how her sensual bravery is making her feel.

Delicate is potent.

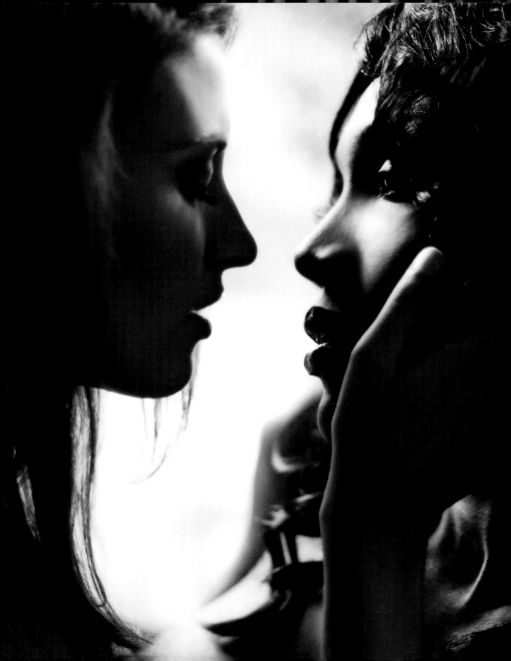

45 Authentic

It's pleasing to play. But she wants to know that **the infatuation is not ephemeral, not lust disguised by love**—that you and she are authentically and enduringly connected.

She places a premium on sincerity, on keeping it real. Without shared values grounded in wisdom and integrity, there can be no harmony.

However, sex and morality often become entangled. False comforts and fake innocence can misshape her moral imagination, leading to inner conflict over seemingly dichotomous parts of herself. She wants to belong, yet strives to stand apart. She values her sexuality, yet feels ashamed about an illicit fantasy that brings her pleasure. The body knows no judgment like the mind does.

Negotiate this paradox, where romance and passion combat the tyranny of reason. Views shouldn't be held too firmly—undo distorted thinking and be realistic in the pursuit of balance and harmony. Live in the more genuine *gray*, rather than the *black and white*.

As her understanding and trust of her sensory nature grows, contradictions remain curious, yet lose their stifling power of dissuasion.

Women want to want. She has a desire to desire—to be free to be.

Encourage her to acknowledge, explore, and celebrate the multiple sides of herself. As a bonus, cognitive dissonance is so psychologically powerful that it often, and quite surprisingly, triggers sexual arousal. And that's **the real deal.**

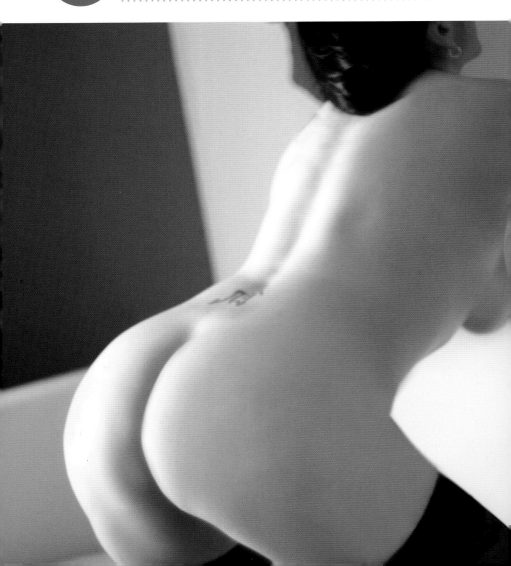

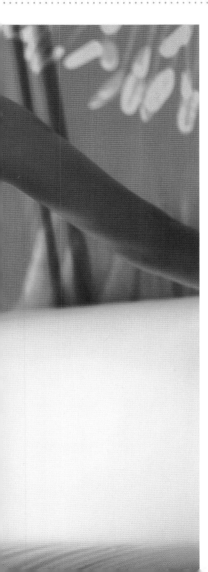

Get down anilingus-style to **please her perky posterior.**

The perineum, a soft, diamond-shaped area in front of the anus extending to the fourchette of the vulva, is an often-neglected treasure that when well attended, relays waves of pleasure messages to her brain.

To intensify her orgasm, massage her *P-spot* by rolling your knuckles along the area. Just before she comes, press into it with your fingertips.

Lick her perineum. Long and slow.

Respect the natural microorganisms in this intimate region. Don't rim bareback. Be smart and safe. Using a latex barrier won't diminish sensations.

Bury your head between her hot fanny cakes to tongue every sensitive groove. *Rimming* is an excellent move to prepare for upcoming penetration, or **a truly satisfying end, in and of itself!**

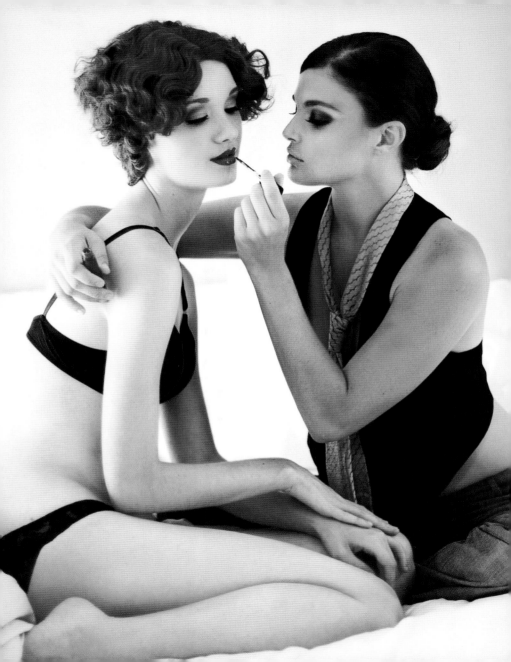

47 Accoutrements

Embody her fantasy.

Throw a decadent, costume-compulsory party to remember.

Revel in the *joie de vivre* of the roaring twenties of New York, London, Paris, and Berlin. Dress in the spirit of Garbo, Crawford, Dietrich, Hepburn, Valentino, Chaplin, Chanel, Mae West, Gertrude and Alice, a flapper or *garçonne*, a suffragist, a surrealist, a gangster, a legendary athlete, or an incomparable muse.

Various eras of history have been **a hotbed of pussy and passion,** indulgence and appreciation, artistic exploration, and sophisticated scene-making.

In the 1920s, new fashions transformed bright young things, who cut their long hair and tossed their corsets to the wind, revealing boyish silhouettes and a newly embraced tough, cool, and seductive nature.

American jazz shook smoky lounges to their core, fueling vital and infectious energy, both creative and erotic.

Dulled sensuality can be sharpened and reinvigorated. Host a sumptuous setting where she's free to celebrate her lust for life without restriction.

Manufacturing her dreams is a juicy business.

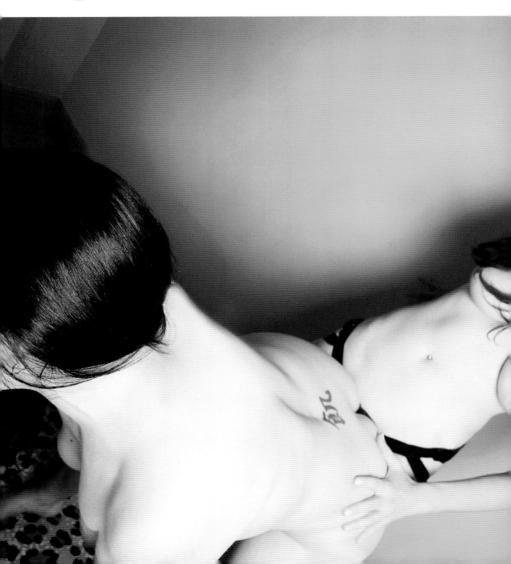

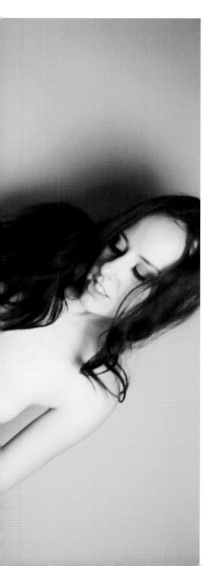

Each woman is a universe. And tools offer an invaluable edge when navigating **her intricate, highly charged galaxy.**

Handywomen don't keep a well-stocked toolbox to replace a lover or raise feelings of inadequacy. *Au contraire*—tools crush limitations, alleviate pressure, and amplify the action.

Since **buzzing onto the scene** in the 1880s, the electric vibrator has doubled as a spare set of lips or superskilled fingers to calm nerves, jump-start arousal, focus a wandering mind, tickle a clit, pass the time, and achieve *plateau* after pleasurable *plateau*.

Wonderful electric!

Innovative gadgets, from simple and stealthy to substantive and adventurous, are constantly being designed—from remote-controlled to waterproof to eco-conscious. Go even greener and include fresh fare: slyly shop the farmers' market for that perfectly shaped, firm cuke.

Support reputable vendors, use lubrication and *rubber johnnies*, follow use and care instructions, and keep your box well stocked.

49 Splosh

Dip me in honey and throw me to the lesbians!

A truly scrumptious way to explore her body is through sexy food play, also known as *sploshing*.

Drizzle her abdomen with sweet, sticky agave nectar. For a more gourmet splosh, mix honey with goat cheese and pureed almonds. Spreading this perfectly gooey concoction on her succulent skin is as much fun as gradually licking it off.

Garnish her breasts with bursts of whipped cream. Top her with swirls of decadent chocolate. **Nourish the passion** that consumes you both and climb aboard.

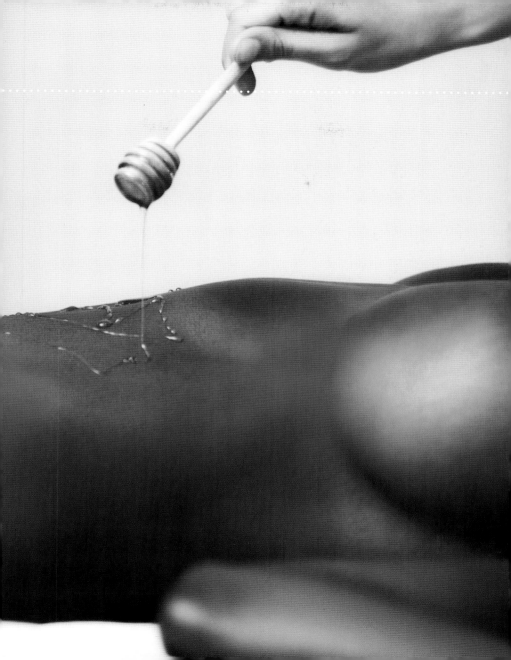

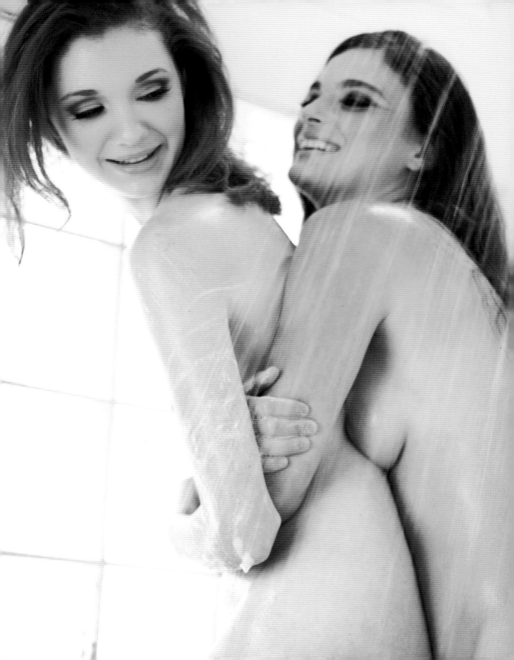

50 Steam

Love, like rain, tears, saliva, and water, is essential to living life. **Intimacy is love's bounty,** yet it's a challenge to make and take time to enjoy it. A solution is to blend intimacy into a routine—shower together.

Saturation is sexy.

Follow the beads of water that travel her contours.

As she lathers herself from head to toe, the light reflecting off her shimmering skin and hair, notice how she systematically touches the different regions of her body, from a gentle caress to aggressive exfoliation. Remember where she lingers.

With a loofah, body sponge, or pouf, especially indulge her hard-to-reach places.

Pursue dual sensations of wetness by kissing her as the water pleasantly pummels you both. Drop to your knees to scrub her buttocks, thighs, shins, calves, and feet.

Alter the setting of the versatile, handheld nozzle—from romantic mists to invigorating pulsations. Target specific areas as she desires. It's a refreshing delight to luxuriate in the shared rewards of an erotic shower.

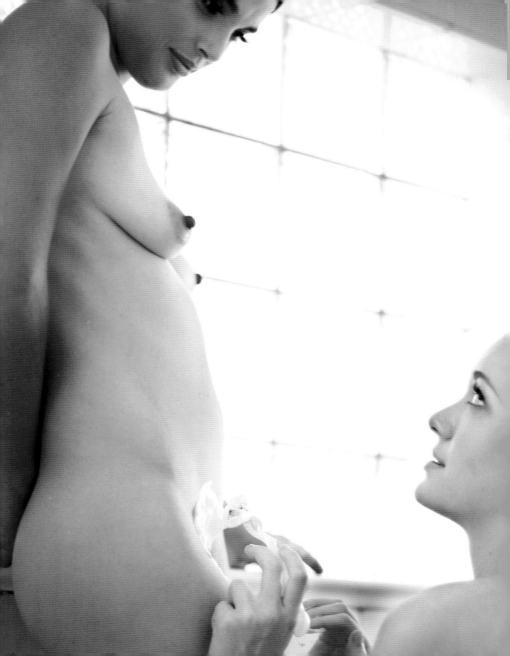

51 Preen

Whether you shave bare, have an eye for design, or primp for exceptional softness, *preen play* is a huge turn-on!

If her desire is to maintain a full bush, share in the adoration and tend her *velvet forest*. Bask in the shower of her pheromones released by your loving care.

Fond of the way it feels or looks, some women choose to shave their armpits, legs, or bush, while others prefer to remain *au naturel*.

Sensually shave her as she lies back on the bed with a towel beneath her, or as she stands in the shower or tub. The anticipation during preparation will trigger sexual thoughts and quickly and visibly arouse her.

Describe what you see and feel, and how you're lovin' it as you **trim her hedges** into a strip or pattern, such as a star or heart. You can also change the hair color with a temporary or permanent dye made especially for **below-the-belt beauty.**

Preen play inevitably leads to pussy play, as your pair of pretty *muffs* are now **all dressed up for someplace to go, go, go.**

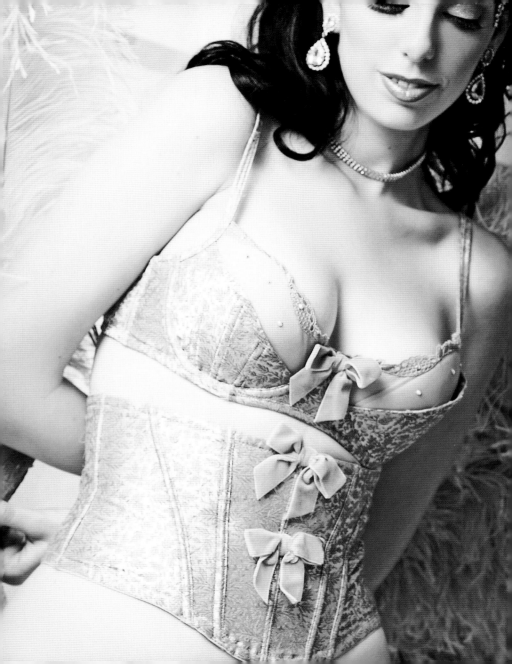

52 Billie's Stopless

Seduce her by proxy.

Treat her to a chic and provocative live performance. Burlesque is a time-honored celebration of bold femininity and sensuality. Take pleasure together in the overt seduction of a high art *bump and grind*!

Typically, she's most affected by what she sees, with the largest majority of her impressions derived from her sense of sight. **Watch her watch** this tantalizing tease. Learn what enthralls her, so that you can gain access to her personal blueprint for stimulation, arousal, and response.

Meld into the mix of devotees. Feed off of the erotic, circulating energy as the smoldering performer struts and poses to titillate and tantalize her fans.

It's an atypical delight to sit together in the shadows and share such a voyeuristic thrill.

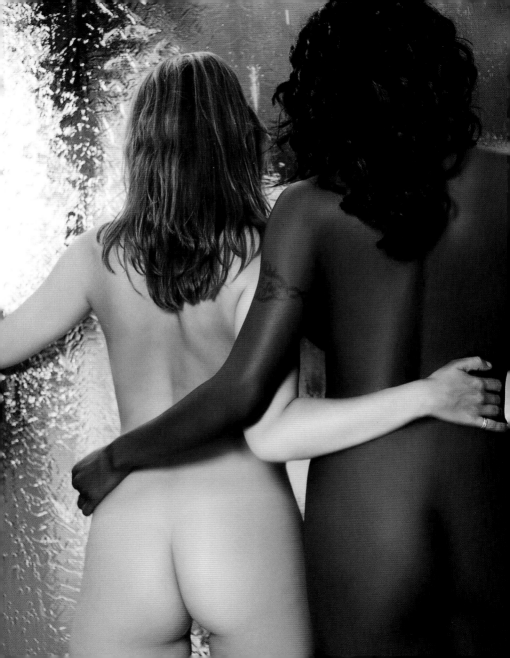

53 Swept Away

Will she run with the big dogs or stay on the porch with the pups?

Life isn't meant to be observed; it's meant to be lived. Embrace a *joie de vivre* for being.

She longs to be swept away. Be her adventurous lover. Pull her off the porch and shatter her routine. Fulfill her dream to explore and experience new worlds.

Her options for adventure are limitless. Immerse yourselves in each other's *destination paradise*.

Step into liquid and surf for the first time. Dive a shipwreck. Sail the river mild. The whoosh and flutter of a hot air balloon flight is sure to lighten her mind, body, and spirit. Gather with bird nerds in picturesque settings to see an elegant eagle soar or a nuthatch scamper up a London plane tree.

Fulfilling her dream adventure, however big or small, gives her the confidence to pursue additional curiosities and passions. It'll also fuel her desire to continue to explore her every passion with you.

Tell her to define her own limits.

Life happens so quickly, my love. Spread your wings today.

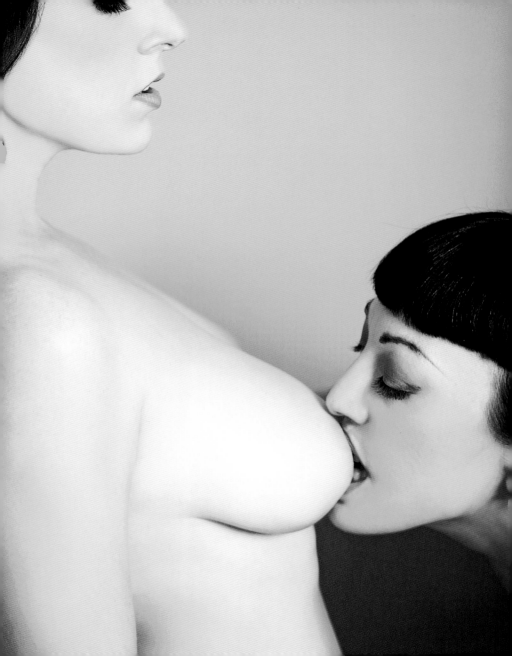

54 Get Her Kink On, Hard

Take her further then she's ever been.

On **the edges of sexuality** lie less conventional practices such as *kink*. As opposed to *fetishism*, in which an object of desire replaces or substitutes for intimacy, kinkiness, which focuses on props and role playing, enhances the closeness of lovers.

Many surfaces offer a sensuous allure. Employ nipple clamps on her nipples to up the erotic ante.

Tease her irresistible nipples until they're erect, firm, and standing proud before gently applying each clip. Give her ample time to respond, mentally and physically—and communicate throughout. Respect the fact that **pleasure and pain are intimate acquaintances,** capable of centering her in or propelling her out of any moment.

Restrict the blood flow to her erect nipples for ten minutes or less. She'll likely endure the most pain not from the initial clamping or from any mild or wild games that ensue, but rather just after tit clip removal.

Youch!

Plus, if she climaxes during clamp play, her nipples will be even more sensitive than usual.

Unclamp one at a time, slowly and with care. Gently lick and suck each tender nipple as the blood rushes back into them and her nerve endings reawaken with fervor.

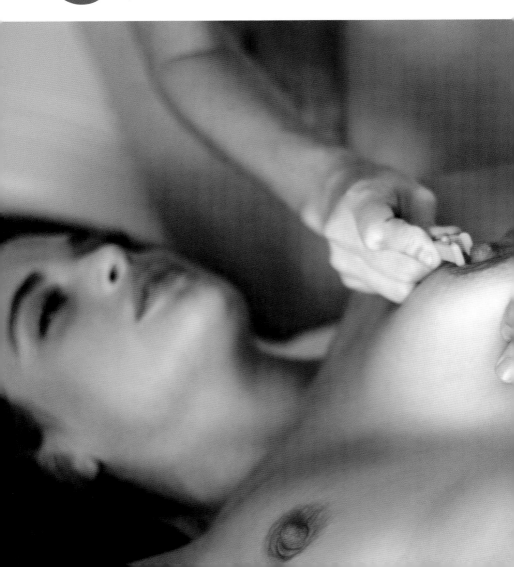

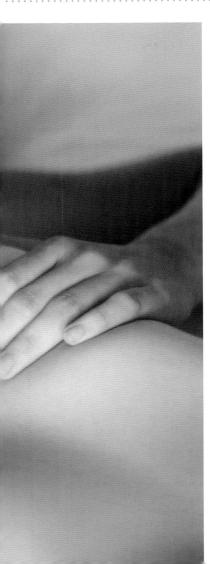

Nipple clamps grant your hands, lips, and tongue a free pass to travel elsewhere. Make the most of the ten minutes during which you have one or both of her lovely nipples clamped.

Turn the *kink* up a notch and simultaneously **tease the tips of her freshly clamped nips** with a flit of your tongue, a soft blush brush, a small vibrator, or even a *shopworn porn* ice cube.

Adjustable clamps offer a lighter or stronger hold, some contain built-in vibrators, and many pairs are joined with a chain to twist and tug with hands or teeth.

Combine clamping with handheld dildo or strap-on sex. **Hold the chain between your teeth for a timely titty tug** each time you thrust into her. And either you or she can control the chain after you transition and enter her from behind.

The same clamps can squeeze her lobes, tongue, any set of lips, underarms, and the backs of the knees to incite a head-to-toe, inside and out, exquisite rush. She'll find the entire experience—and you—bracing as she revels in **a perfect mix of peril and pleasure.**

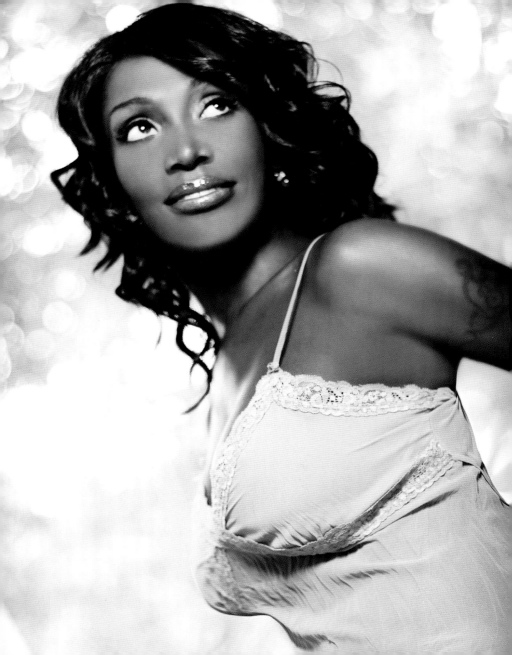

56 Salut d'Amour

She wants you on your knees.

It may be a well-worn tradition, yet one would be hard-pressed to dispute how deeply affecting this romantic gesture can be.

Through touch, you and she simultaneously receive, transmit, and share your feelings. Take her hand in yours, lift it to your lips, and kiss her hand with tenderness.

Drop to one knee, look deeply into her eyes, and proclaim your intentions, adoration, and undying love.

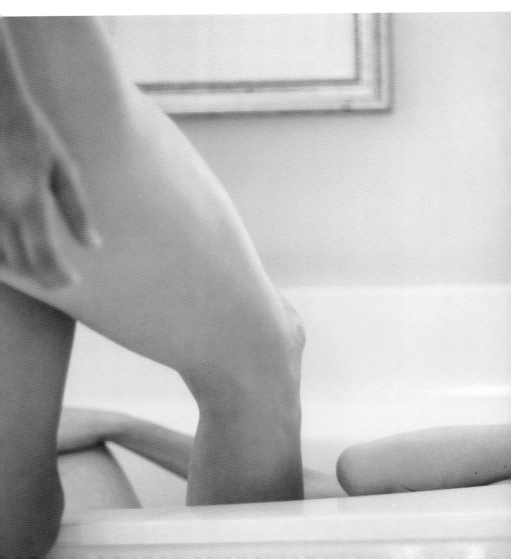

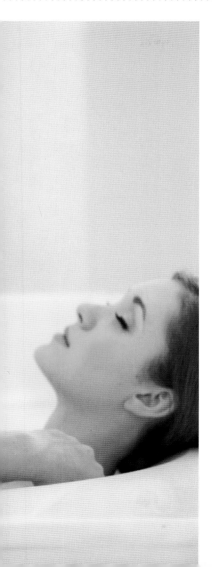

Sexiness is a state of mind, body, and soul.

Establish consistent places of calm amid the hustle and flow where each of you can replenish, restore, and strengthen your core.

To get out of your head, you have to get into it. Meditation, yoga, and tai chi teach practitioners to properly breathe, relax, and release. Explore these practices to expand your potential to know greater peace, significance, interconnectedness, and fulfillment.

When **mentally and physically supple,** you and she can focus on the sublime and sensual in all things.

The pursuit of wellness will also enhance your abilities to express the awesome potency of your divine feminine sexuality. It's a **passion payoff** for you both when you summon your renewed sensual essences to rise and collide.

Onward and upward!

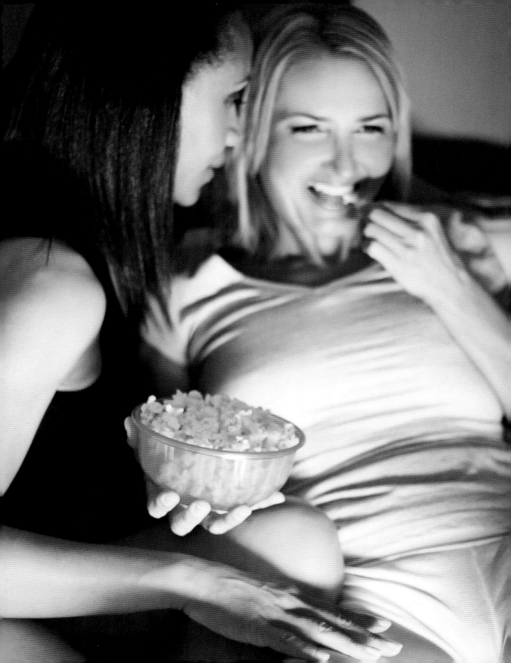

58 Popcorn and Porn

By recent estimates, one in three **women watch erotica,** alone and with friends and lovers.

She can allow her imagination free rein to identify with the characters, scenarios, and on-screen action, or can simply bask in the sexy mood. Observing often proves to be a stirring segue into participating in your own steamy storyline.

Fool around while a blue movie flickers in the background.

Let her watch while you sexually pleasure her.

Rent or buy. Test the waters by ordering a short clip on demand.

Erotic movies have come a long way. The abundance of genres include fantasy, kinky, fetish, how-to's, multicultural, foreign, art, butch, femme, reality, LGBTI (lesbian, gay, bisexual, transgender, intersex), soft-core, hard-core, hetero, and by women for women.

Enthusiasts of erotica or porn don't necessarily want to do the things they see. In fact, **embracing the outrageousness is often quite grounding.** And when she feels grounded, she'll be more at ease about flaunting each and every sensual side of herself.

At the end of the day, **as the credits roll, it's still all about love.**

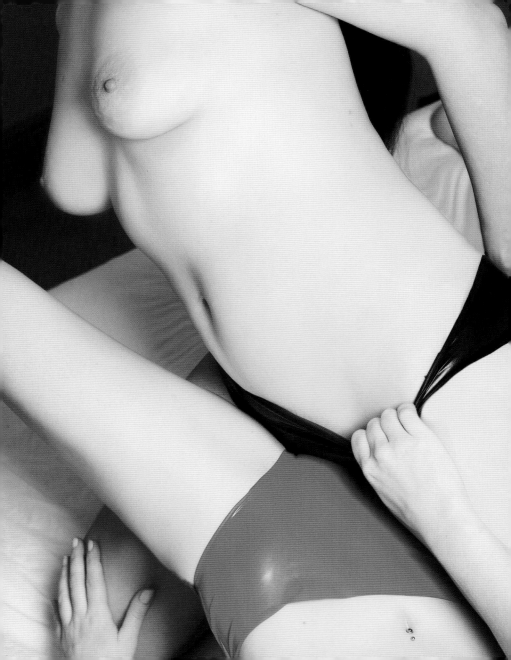

59 Artifice

Adorn her body with latex, a sexy gimmick with extraordinary visual and tactile dimensions.

Use latex body paints to brush a glittery clubbing outfit, lingerie, or a superheroine or villain disguise onto her skin. Explore a fantasy that inspires both the artist and her muse.

Latex, which is rubber suspended in water, evolved out of the pursuit for a better condom. Its strength and outstanding elastic qualities inspires many uses and designs, from kinky to vanilla.

Squeeze into *ready-to-wear* latex fashions. **The tightness is a tantalizing taste of sexual bondage** for you both as the latex grips your bodies.

Deliver extra heat to your aroused *la-las* by mashing your latex-encased pussies together.

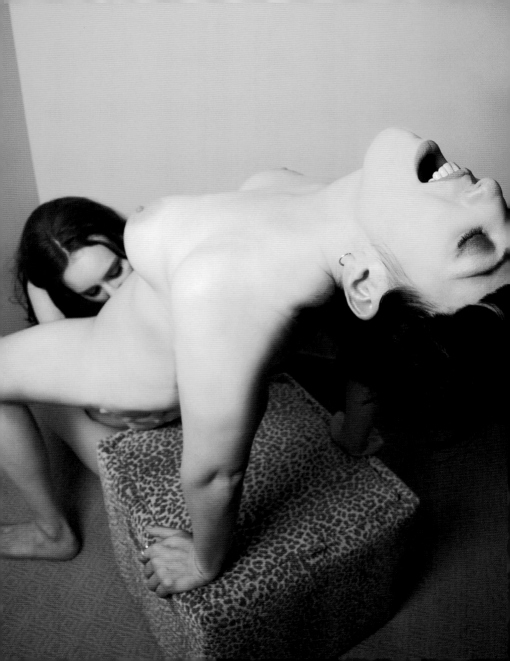

60 On the Edge of Her Seat

Make your move to **scandalize her when she's sitting unaware in a chair.**

Place your hands on her hips, and then scoot her to the edge of her seat. Mischievously lift her skirt or undo and remove her pants. Touch her through her panties and exhale a gentle breath of warm air onto *her flower.*

Pull her panties off, and proceed with an impromptu session of oral pleasure. Lift her hips slightly when she's about to climax—by clenching her surprisingly sensitive gluteus muscles as she comes, her orgasm will be super-*maximus.*

If her chair offers the advantage of mobility, create some unconventional amusement park thrills. Hold your head still while swiveling her chair to and fro. She'll giggle with a growing giddiness each time your tongue pushes her clit's button and **her pussy sweeps across the length of your industrious lips.**

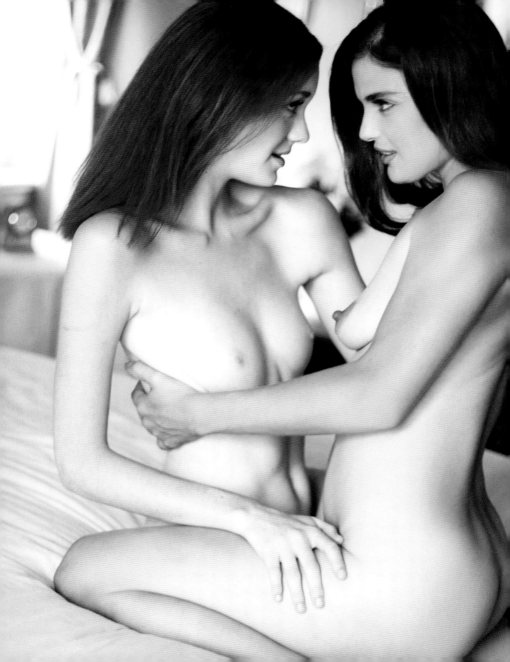

61 Just Fuckin'

Yesterday is history. Tomorrow's a mystery.

Let her get out of her head and feel.

Sex is not always an expression of love. **Plunge into your carnal natures.** The further you and she can simultaneously move beyond your minds, the more **raw and sensorially rich** your sexual connection will be.

Get oozingly messy with messin' around that's about **nuthin' but the fuckin'.** No plan, no prelude, and no talk beyond murmuring an inclination or hot spot to pleasure—just two voracious women having **high-octane sex** on instinct.

Never begrudge your lover her urges and appetites. And never take the familiar and accessible for granted.

Fuck good, always.

62 Gushing

Experience the marvel of female ejaculation.

A woman may remarkably expel fluid of a unique chemical composition through her urethra just before or during her orgasm. Most often, these *waterworks* occur when her G-spot is aroused. An open vaginal canal is usually required to expel this love juice; she'll emit it once you withdraw a sex toy or your fingers.

For most women, this transparent, warm, viscous, aromatic fluid releases about a teaspoon of involuntary drip. A woman highly skilled at this showy display can voluntarily ejaculate, **gushing with pleasure for her astonished lover.**

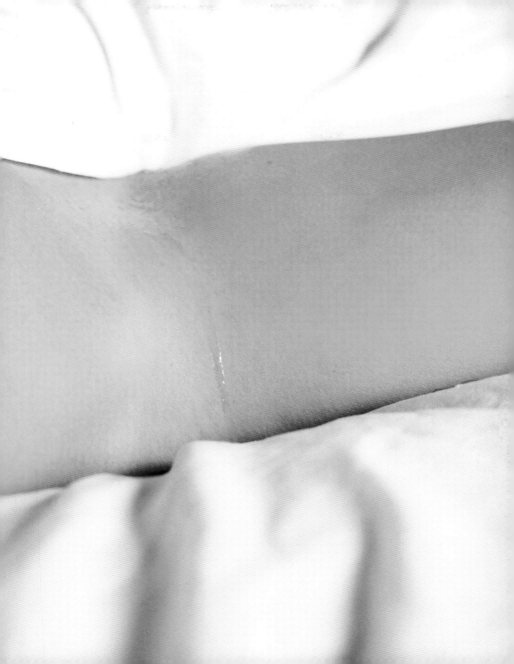

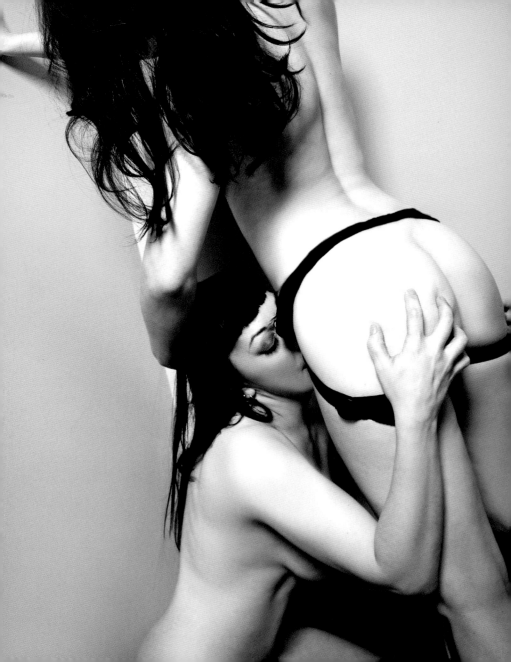

63 Suck Off

The visual impact is stunning. But the pressure alone from a good **girl-on-girl blow job,** also known as *stud muffin'*, will *untangle her tingle* every time for a phenomenal mental and clitoral climax.

Before she fucks you with the *strap-on clit extension* she's prancing around in, a remarkable way to ignite both familiar and unfamiliar sensations is to **give her head.**

Power is an indisputable aphrodisiac.

Suck her off as she watches from above, submitting to and feeding the illusion.

Begin with enthusiastic *lip service*, licking the length of *her member*. As you hit upon the rhythm, the head moving in and out of your mouth, authoritatively stroke the shaft to enliven the show. Keep one hand on the base to control the depth of motion. Press the base into her pussy to meet her clit on every plunge.

A vibrator strategically placed under or in the pocket of her harness adds constant stimulation to amplify her odds of climaxing while she's being blown.

For the *finale royale*, coddle and squeeze her clit extension in your glistening cleavage, and **fuck her raging hard-on with your titties.**

Your lubricated finger slipping into her ass just as she's nearing climax will skyrocket this already euphoric woman to a jaw-dropping altitude!

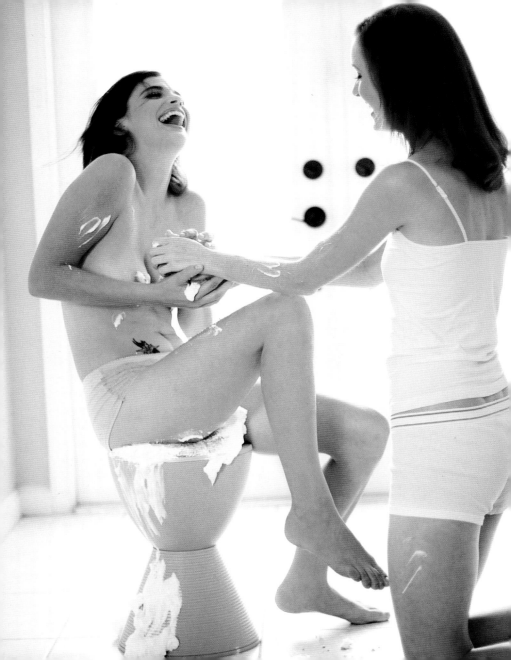

64 Pie-Sexual

Sweet dreams are made of this.

Sometimes she takes it all too seriously. Keep it real by playfully capitalizing on her vulnerability. Shock her sense of decorum and **temporarily defile her beauty with a sweet and sticky surprise.**

Buy a graham cracker crust, and then make your own filling—grocery pies tend to be heavy in consistency. Fill it with chocolate, banana, or whipped cream. Add sexy toppings, such as caramel or berry sauce to taste.

The fascination with *pie play* dates back to silent movie slapstick. Concoct a time-honored sneak attack during which your babe in the woods becomes the viscous victim of a classic *pieing*.

Or pretend the creaming is an accident. As you permit her to dip her finger into the mixing bowl, the thought won't cross her sweetly naive mind that you intend anything other than serving up a thoughtful, yummy dessert. Then cream her!

Wipe, lick, and kiss off the remnants as an additional *skirmish* unfolds from this **fresh foreplay full of messy giggles.**

She's thrilled to have a lover who is the perfect blend of angel and devil.

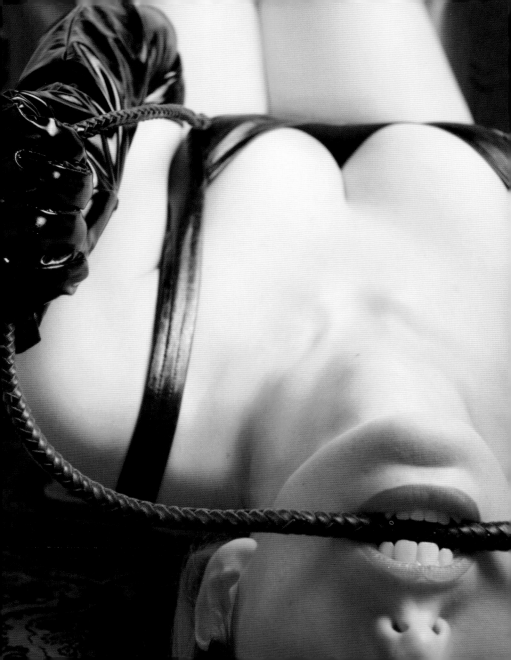

65 Who's on Top?

Give her an inch and she thinks she's a ruler. Power is intoxicating.

Women's attributes, goals, and dreams vary greatly. Yet all women alternately lead and follow, are vulnerable and powerful, in some way every day. When you exhibit control, she loses hers.

Boldness is incredibly sexy. **Dominate her.** When she relinquishes authority, she'll know the pleasure found in surrender.

A naughty submissive may feign disrespect and test boundaries. Exclusive of her engaging a *safe word* to halt everything, your wish remains her command.

Control the momentum. Be persuasive as you assert your power in this safe zone of erotic fantasy.

Be mild or wild as you take control.

The role of even a casual mistress leading a light, at-home game of *cat with a whip and mouse* requires stamina—physical and mental—to keep the experience progressive and focused. There are **many ways to top your bottom in this mysterious space where body and mind merge.** Immerse to escape.

The powerlessness she feels in the presence of your commanding vitality intrigues her.

Powerlessness is the energy that fuels her desire.

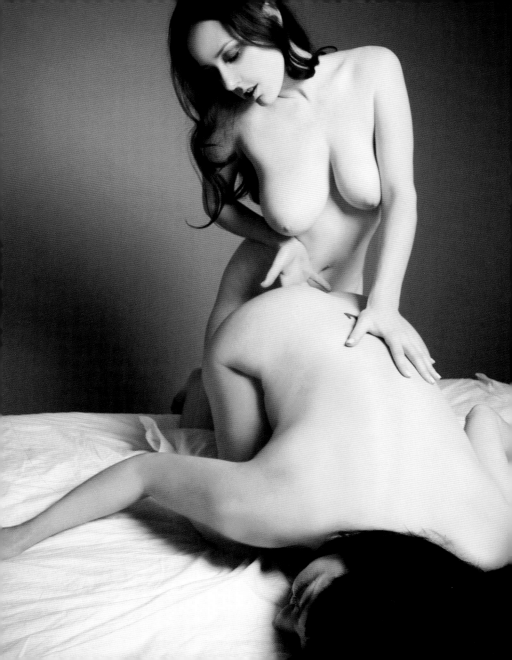

66 Gamble and "Proct" Her

Release her *puckering starfish* and slip inside.

Many women are astonished to discover that they prefer anal to vaginal penetration. The deeply felt, unique sensations can lead her to know unprecedented sexual pleasure.

As with the clitoris and labia, blood rushes to the scores of nerve endings in this region when it's aroused. Once excited, the rectum dilates in anticipation of further consideration.

Take it slowly. Don't surprise her with a sudden attempt to enter her *booty*; she must be well prepared, both mentally and physically, for this **naughty and delicate act** that teeters on the precipice of pain and pleasure. Little natural lubricant is produced by the membrane in this particular erogenous zone, so lube up generously for all forms of play.

Slip a finger or an ass-specific toy inside. Her preferred depth of penetration is subjective and will vary from encounter to encounter. Ongoing communication, safe and clean behavior, perceptive adjustments, and practice will make perfect.

To change it up, stimulate her with a small vibrator at the point of entry.

Once you're inside and she's comfortable, drive her completely wild with your free hand by **drumming her ready and waiting clitoris** with your fingertips and intermittently slapping her sweet ass.

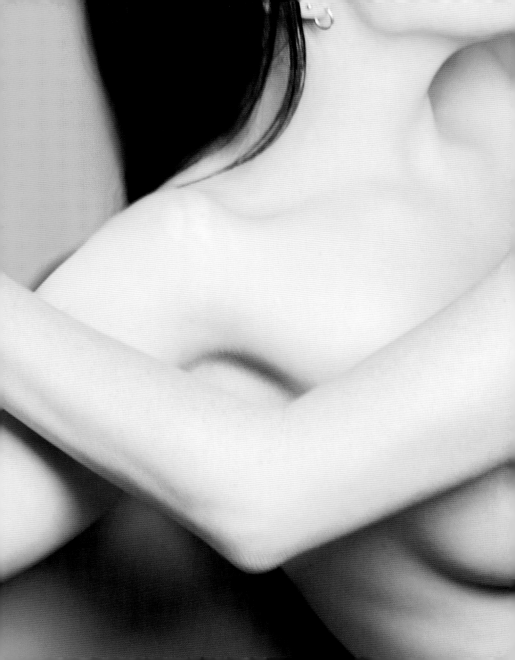

67 Submission

Everyday life is limiting.

Clear her channel with pure escapism. Pleasant diversions distract and dissolve inhibitions, allowing desires to surface. A life-altering transformation is not elusive, and can come from a newly realized wish.

Lovers in successful relationships **surrender to each other,** and who's on top turns on a dime. Experiment with **the other side of the proverbial paddle** and submit to her say-so.

Passive is exciting.

Sharing power is a challenge, as is refraining from reciprocation during sex. Show her how you trust her with your willingness to be cuffed or blindfolded.

Counterbalance compliance with gestures of hesitation to create and build tension. Her lust for you—and for this pleasurable and perhaps uncharacteristic display of dominance—will be intensified when she sees and feels you truly surrender to her command.

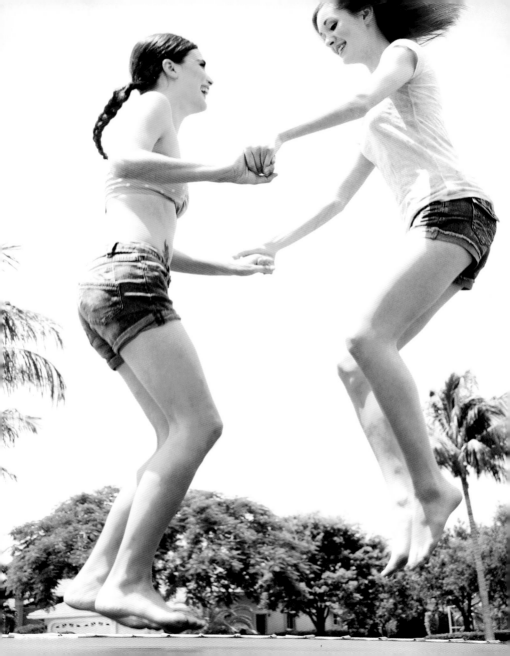

68 Salad Days

Devolve.

Bare your adolescent heart, and **disarm her with your exuberance.**

Be unpretentious, without cynicism, and unburdened.

Think and act unconventionally, maintaining a blissful, willful ignorance of convention.

A ride on a Ferris wheel is enchanting. Side by side, around and around, live in the moment as you slowly take in the unique perspective. Giggle delightedly and squeeze her knee when your heart skips a beat for that brief, giddy instant when the wheel moves past its topmost point and begins its descent—when all you're aware of are two pairs of dangling legs, powerlessly suspended above the earth.

Permit yourself to be silly. Unabashedly refuse to act your age. **The world is your playground.**

Tangle her up with a round of Twister. Take her on in Indian leg wrestling, the feel and smell of the cool, spring grass enveloping you both as you roll around atop its buoyant blades.

Play tag with the neighborhood kids. Be *it*.

Joy liberates.

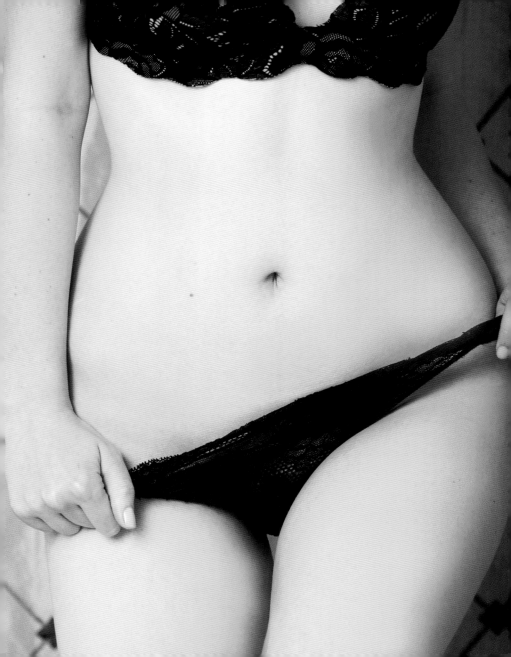

69 Shake Your Booty

Channel your inner exhibitionist.

Entice her sweet spot with a mischievous visual seduction.
A striptease has timeless allure.

The best tease is subtle. Take your time to unclasp, unzip, and unveil.
Playfully **offer her a peek of your pie** before covering the goods
and removing something else. Invite her to participate and begin to
remove her clothing as well.

Costumes and props are optional and limitless. Ignite her glitter fetish
with something that shimmers. Reveal new lingerie under your day-to-
day duds. Go into character and be bawdy, or innocent, or a cop.

Choose music that meshes with your style and rhythmic abilities.
Practice in front of a mirror to shed apprehensions. Show her how you
love to entertain and turn her on.

Above all, have fun taking it all off! She's not awaiting an expert tassel
twirl or pole move. An enthusiastic amateur is very, very sexy.

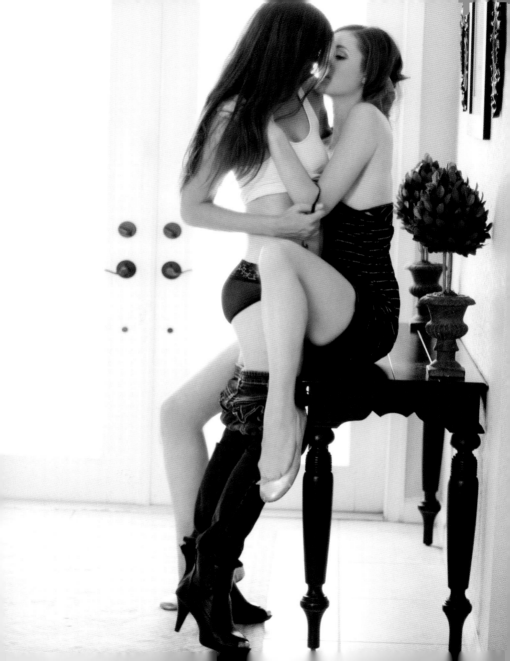

70 Quickie on Cue

Instant gratification is largely undervalued. It's the savvy lovers—those familiar with how pleasurably immediate rewards can linger—who seize every opportunity to perform a *quickie on cue*.

In the last-minute preparations before a dinner party, moments before your guests arrive, boost your stunning co-hostess onto the perfectly set, crystal-laden table, hike up her dress, and get it on.

Unexpectedly lock your office door and ravage her on your desk. Inform the inquisitive salesperson

I'm just looking for my friend

as you slip into her dressing room and slide your hand down her pants.

Lovers pulsate with an incredible sense of urgency. Struggle to keep quiet as you virtually tear off each other's clothes in the throes of passion, **so nearly exposed.** As in a spirited game of hide-and-seek, **the thrill is in the possibility of discovery.**

Bond over building a romantic portfolio of daring, illicit acts and encounters blindly launched and guided by desire. It's exhilarating to misbehave.

Naughty behavior favorably spikes sex hormones, but does little for orgasmic concentration. For your next delirious romp, focus the energy that's sweeping through her body—pull her panties to the side and press a portable vibrator onto her clitoris to swiftly *launch her rocket.*

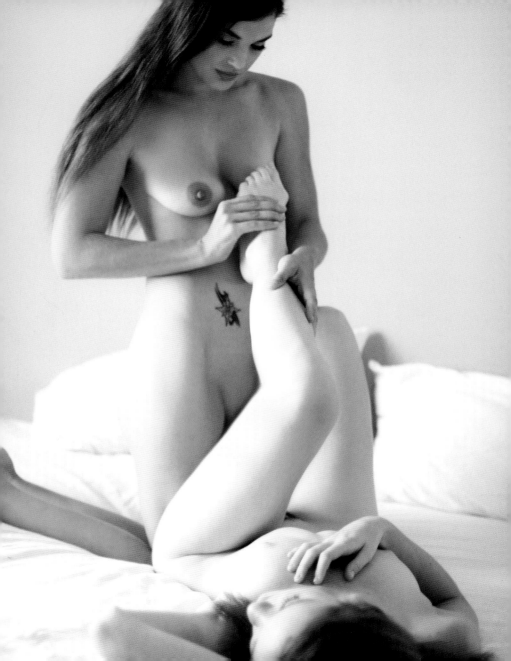

71 Her Dogs Are Barking

Feet are consistently neglected, even though the benefits of attending to these sensual powerhouses are plentiful.

Touch her from sole to soul. Rub her feet to alleviate tension, heal and rejuvenate her from the bottom up, and build her overall resilience.

Often called the body's second heart, feet have more nerve endings than the back and legs combined. Press and hold specific points to unblock her vital life force energy pathways.

Warm cream or an herbal oil in your hands and then caress her calves, encircle her ankles with your thumbs, grip and squeeze her soles, and knead the contours of her arches.

Press one foot onto your breast, resting her heel within your cleavage as you pamper her other foot. Her body loves symmetrical attention.

The transmission hubs in the brain for the feet and the clitoris are adjacent. Therefore, it's highly likely that her tootsies and her clit partake in pillow talk, gleefully swapping sensual information.

Happy feet, happy pussy!

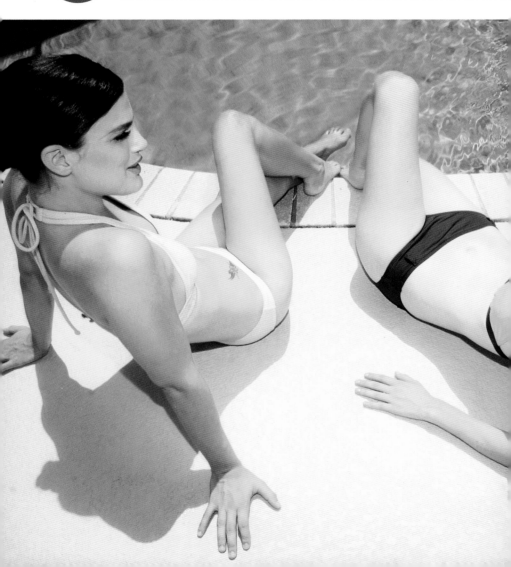

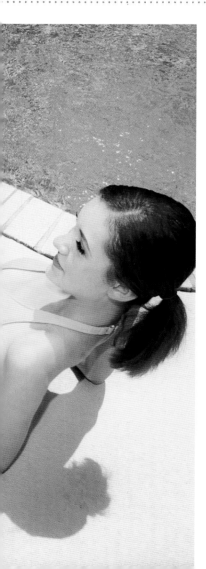

She says I never listen to her.
At least, I think that's what she says.

It's her wish to be heard, considered, and understood. *Hear* her spoken and unspoken messages, ponder their implications and intentions, and succinctly and thoughtfully respond.

An ultimate joy for her is to interact with a considerate and captivated listener.

To truly hear also involves hearing within yourself the insights and yearnings that are worthy of expression.

Shooting the breeze passes the time—but you're talking into the wind. Deepen your understanding of the world with spirited conversations of substance. These exchanges forge the strongest connections and bring you both the most pleasure and fulfillment.

Mutual mental gymnastics will also create an abundance of cherished memories to everlastingly **stir her mind, her heart, and her chamber of Venus.**

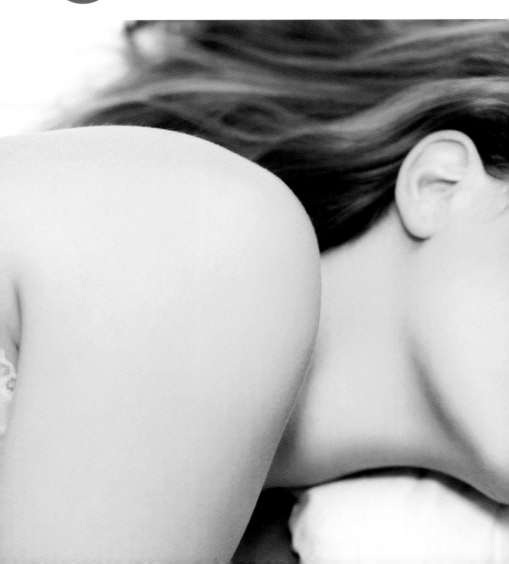

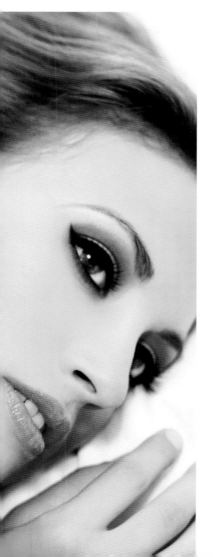

Wherever you go, there you are. Take pleasure in your own company. A woman's best friend is herself.

As a relationship matures, it's important to preserve individuality. Pursue your own hobbies, kicks, and thrills, and encourage her to do the same.

Happiness is mostly a choice. It's far from the easiest choice, and being happy requires constant cultivation. Invest in your own happiness in order to bring strength, joy, and energy to your relationship. **Cherish her by valuing and nurturing your own distinctiveness.**

Inspiration is often drawn from reflection. Get away for an occasional weekend or retreat alone. She can **yearn for your return** only if you're not around.

Intermittently withdraw to separate spaces to help maintain a balance between intimacy and autonomy.

Sleep apart. Separate bedchambers can incite a number of steamy role-play scenarios . . .

Hello, room service?

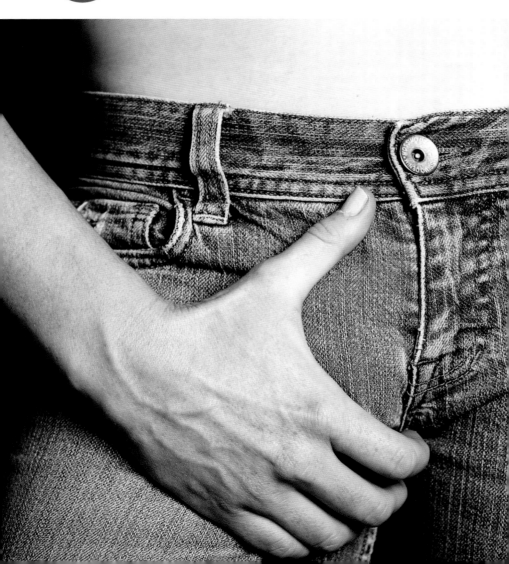

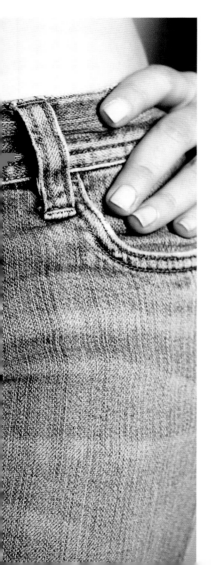

Declare **Clit Awareness Day** and spend it *packin'*!

For hundreds of years, Ben Wa or Geisha balls have been inserted into the vagina or anus to exercise the Kegel muscles and enhance stimulation. Sensual supplements evolve, and a range of kinky complements are available to any woman with a desire to *pack*.

Rebels with a cause refuse to be marginalized. **Gender bending** shatters boundaries. Position your individual packages inside your undies and become familiar—touch, squeeze, stroke, move about, check angles in the mirror, and rearrange accordingly.

Surreptitiously commute, work, shop, dine, and exercise with your precious packages in place.

The interplay of her clit, its accessory, and her mind transforms her attitude. Usually hidden in her labial folds, her *natural pleasure hub* is now in constant contact with a new playmate. She'll be delighted and empowered as **clitoral awareness is gloriously thrust** into the forefront of her consciousness.

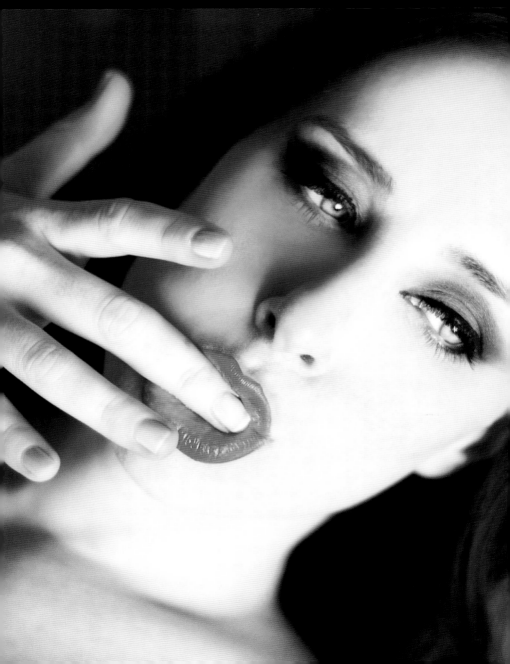

75 Have Cake; Will Eat It, Too

Make her your partner in a crime of extravagance. Indulgence in a forbidden passion is a delicious way to connect.

Dark chocolate contains the amino acid phenylethylamine, a neurotransmitter that raises the body's endorphin levels, elevating her outlook and lifting her libido. The chemical dopamine is subsequently released in the pleasure center of the brain, a reward hub that lights up when something is enjoyable, and then boosts her desire to repeat the behavior and keep the pleasure flowing.

Because chocolate has the power to both stimulate and satiate sexual appetite, save the treat until after the loving. Sensitivities are heightened after sexual activity, so whatever she smells, tastes, feels, and hears will then be more compelling and succulent.

Cater to her *petite praline*. Then unveil an exotic chocolate sampler with an accompanying flight of wines or teas. The melting point of cocoa butter is just below body temperature. The guilty pleasure that you press between her lips will literally **melt in her mouth.**

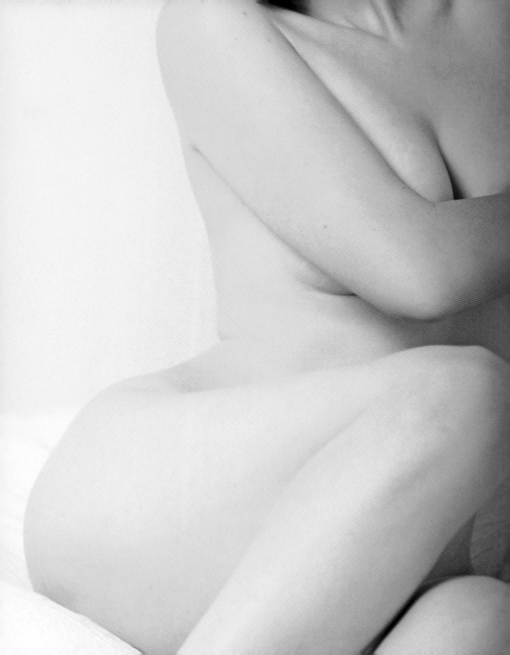

76 Abstain

Champagne is not for every day.

Extraordinary pleasures are to be looked forward to and cherished.

Likely, the two of you have been fucking like bunnies every day since you first came together.

Practice restraint (which, in this context, is not a reference to bondage play).

A brief breather from getting **hot, heavy, and sexually high** on each other creates opportunities to affirm that the two of you share a soul-nurturing bond.

Abstaining from sex is also a delicious game of mounting anticipation—thinking about sex can truly be as much fun as having it.

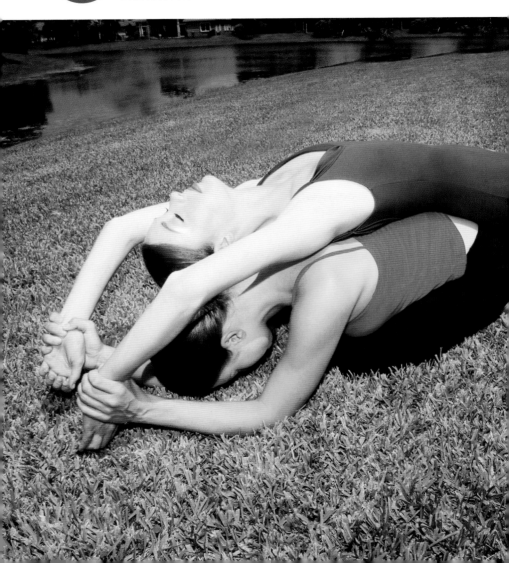

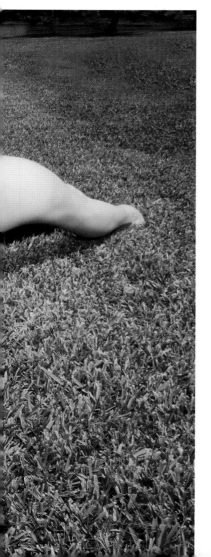

Lithely and lovingly lift and lower the long leg of your limber lover. Yoga, which means *union* in Sanskrit, can unite your body, mind, and spirit with hers.

There's much **beauty and grace** in shared movement. As your bodies engage, admire their features and span.

Experiment with a range of postures like forward folds, backbends, twists, and inversions. Breathe deeply and constantly. Listen to your bodies and respect limits as abilities grow.

Whether a prolonged, gentle stretch or one of intense exertion, you and she will unblock energy, release tense muscles, enhance agility, build strength and stamina, heighten body awareness and control, and boost your moods, capacities, and likelihood for sexual pleasure.

Keep stretch bands, a cushy mat, and an inflatable physio ball nearby—this equipment is indispensable when your partner yoga unfolds into a playful and passionate session of *pussy pilates*.

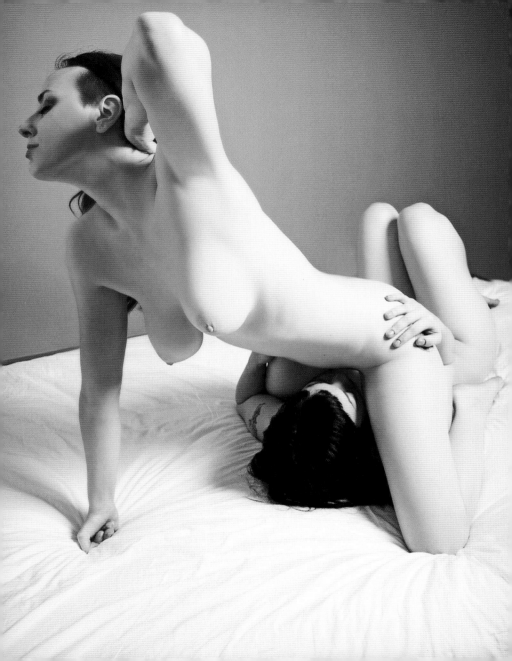

78 Fur-Lined Teacup

Straddling is a form of embrace with a dash of possession. Kneel over her, teasing her with your inviting pussy that floats above her, just out of reach, until she insistently grips your hips and pulls you to her lips.

Lift and lower yourself to control the tastes of pleasure. **Shifts and swings in power are exciting.**

Lower and press your clit into her face when you want it harder; rise again to ease the action.

While she *polishes your jewels*, fondle her breasts, or collide with her fingers and tongue as you dip in to feel and perhaps taste yourself.

With your warm wetness on her mouth, her hips wriggle about as *her flower* also swells with excitement. Without disrupting the mouth-on-pussy contact, lean back and feel her arousal. She may insist that you focus solely on the *lip service* she's dishing out. If she allows mutual pleasuring to continue, consider transitioning so that you can simultaneously **sip each other's sweet tea.**

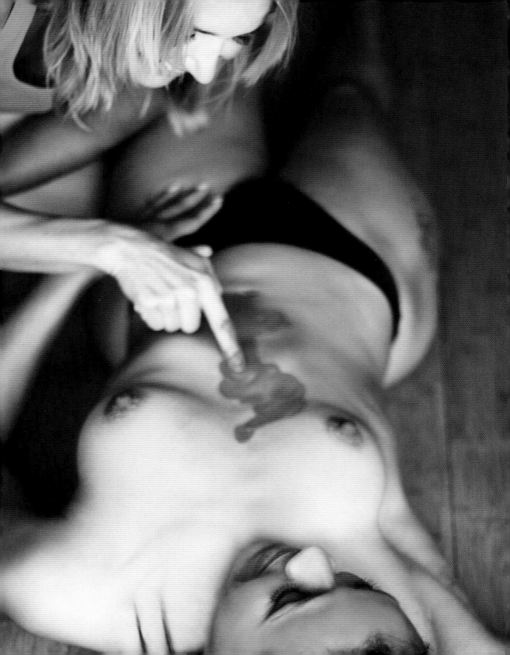

79 Written on the Body

Paint her mountain, gild her nipples, and color the river that leads to *her ocean.*

Her body is your canvas.

A particularly sensuous way to appreciate the contours of her body is to apply color and texture along her lines—every captivating crevice and luscious curve.

Using the sediment from a fifteen-year-old tawny port, fingerpaint a work of art across her midriff.

Encourage her to guess each amusing or risqué cipher you map out on her smooth skin. Scrawl your messages of adoration backward to have fun with mirrors. Leave a reminder on her so that the next day, when she fondles it as she might a favorite bracelet, she'll think of you.

Variety is the spice of sex, and body paints come in an assortment of colors, scents, and tastes for you to realize any motif that she inspires.

There are so many ways to **touch her glittering garden.**

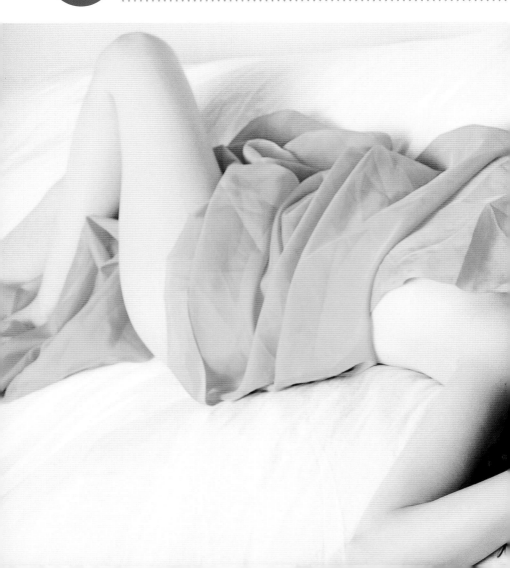

and Last

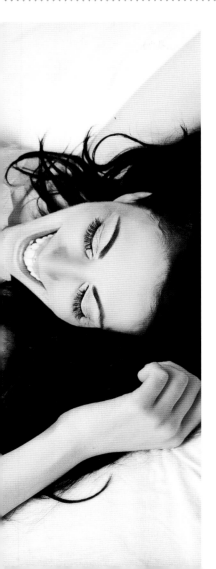

Her clit will not be kept down.

After a climax, a woman is often ripe for more, and may in fact experience several ecstatic rushes of orgasmic pleasure with little recovery time in between.

Her seismic sequels to the first installment will usually be more intense and far-reaching.

After her first orgasm, briefly direct attention away from her supersensitive swollen *bud*. Let your fingers and mouth **joyride inside her velvet folds.** Detour along her perineum or to her breasts before returning to slow, feather-light licks across her hedonistic *princess in a boat*.

When you prolong your sexcapades, whether or not you experience the thrilling phenomenon of multiple orgasms, your mutual production of endorphins increases—a collaborative creation of **round-the-clock euphoria.**

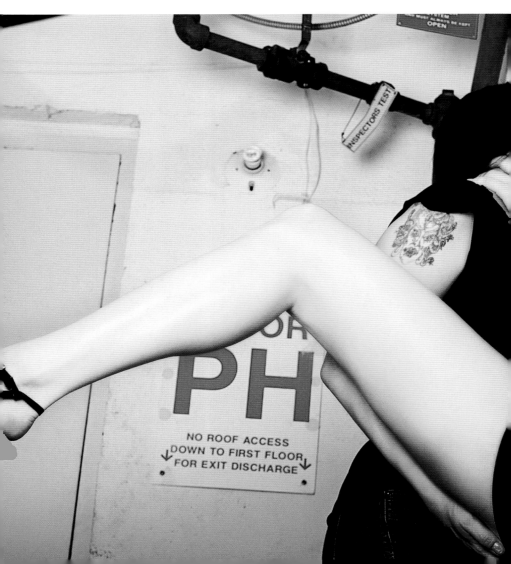

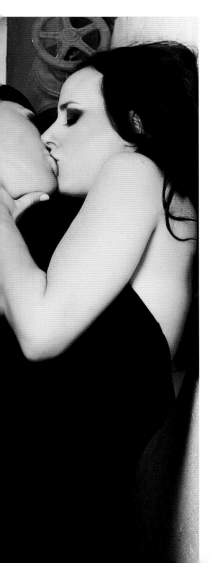

A zipless fuck.

This provocative phrase, infamously coined by Erica Jong in *Fear of Flying*, describes a longing for a sexual encounter with a stranger that is purely for its own sake—no ties, expectations, or agendas beyond loveless sexual pleasure.

Oscar Wilde declared illusion to be *the first of all pleasures.* Disguising reality stimulates her brain and has an exhilarating ripple effect on her body. Much of the appeal of this powerful *zipless* hookup fantasy is the opportunity to **be uninhibited without judgment.**

Arrange to slip away with her for an *anonymous* tryst. Meet, bolt into unbridled sex, climax or don't, then exit separately.

Maintain the illusion and forever share a dirty little secret by never breaking character. She'll delight in reliving the encounter during future pillow talk, when you reveal the intimate details of a **thrilling rendezvous** you once had with an incredible *exotic stranger.*

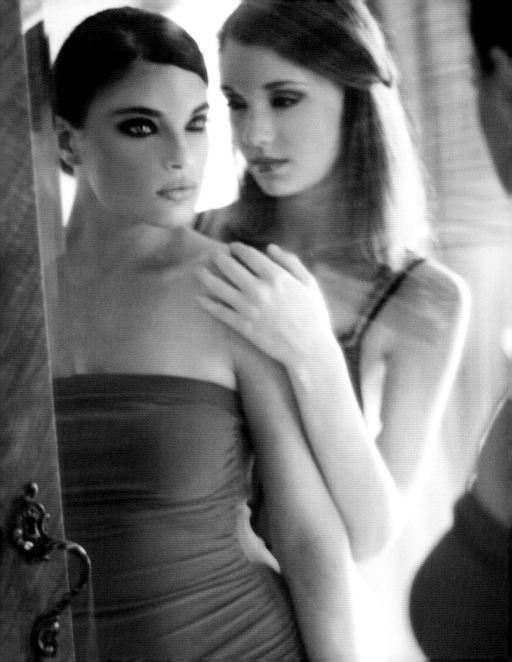

82 Mind over Matter

She may have been attracted to your sparkling eyes, supple skin, rock-hard thighs, or kiss-me-now lips, but she'll fall in love with your intelligence, humor, vision, and generosity.

The depth of your attractiveness has to do with your mind-set and what you're doing with your talents, gifts, and opportunities.

We're all just passengers on the time train. Random acts of kindness have an astonishingly widespread transformative effect.

Einstein declared, *a life lived for others is the only life worth living.* Benevolence is **an intoxicating tonic for the soul.** The need to do good is as fundamental as food, and the satisfaction derived is as primal a human pleasure as sex.

Humility and generosity are equally sexy. Touch a life and make a difference in your own way.

Impress her by virtue of your character. The woman to whom she'll *hitch her wagon* must be an expression of a finer part of herself.

Be the woman with whom she'll share all aspects of her life, privately and socially, including her every need, desire, and sensual pleasure. **It's from shared admiration that deeper love grows.**

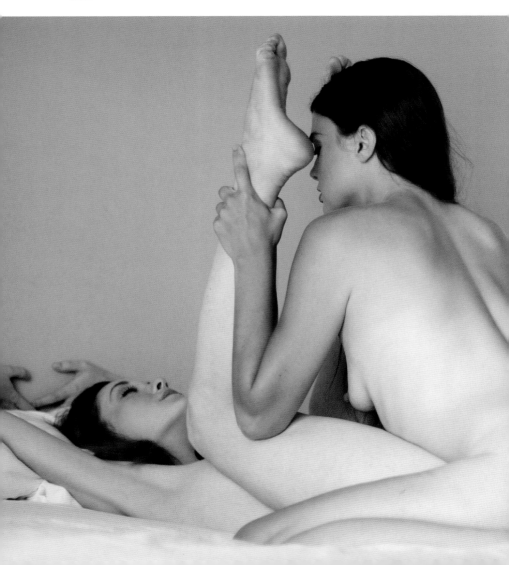

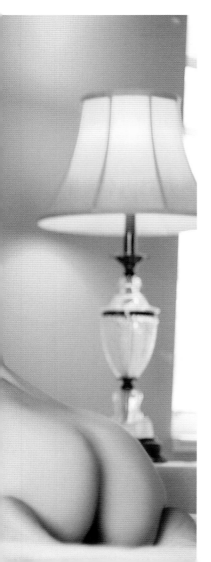

Lovers thrust their hips and pound their pelvises together to intensify arousal, express lust, and deepen all connections. Everyday sex maintains its stronghold when you transgress the parameters of *vanilla*.

Sit on and straddle her, and before entering her, send her out of bounds by caressing her lips with your *nips*.

During sex, grab each other's nipples and squeeze in sync with each driving force.

When she's below, she'll feel you **penetrate her more deeply** when she draws her knees up to her chest and hugs them, or raises her legs and rests her feet on your chest or drapes them over your shoulders. **For the tightest fit,** keep her legs as straight and elevated as possible.

As you fuck her with your fingers or a sex accessory, clasp onto her ass, pull her in to you, embrace her, and savor the breadth of your skin-on-skin contact. **Freeze-frame a thrust,** staying inside her as you stimulate your clitoris until you orgasm. Releasing and clenching her pulsating pussy as she awaits her turn to climax, **she's buzzing and blissfully breathless.**

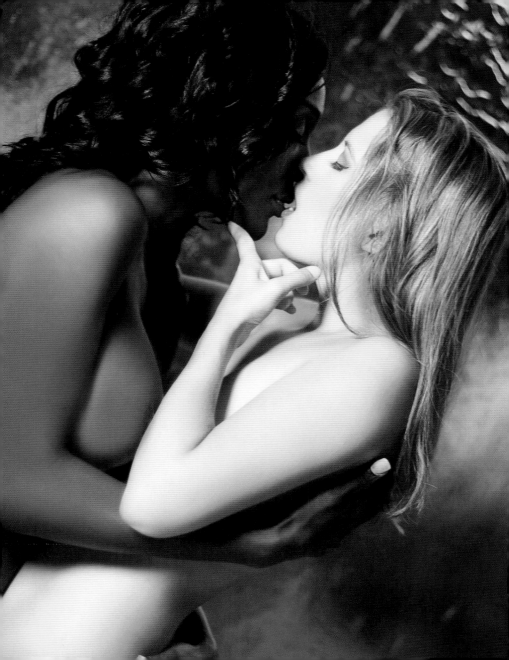

84 Mouth to Mouth

The essence of French kissing is in **the meeting of tongues.**

The best kisser never bumps her partner's nose or teeth, is an avid reader of body language, responds, and reciprocates. She knows that her mighty tongue is an impressive collection of muscles covered with thousands of highly sensitive receptors capable of inducing appetite and enhancing pleasure.

Moisten your lips with a light brush of your tongue before pressing them against hers. Close your eyes and take your time as intimacy is lost on those who rush.

As you kiss, part your lips slightly and slowly run the tip of your tongue along her lips, **nudging her to welcome you inside.**

Inhale her breath and draw in her essence as you slowly enter her with a soft and supple tongue. Gently touch and playfully twirl your tongue with hers.

As you continue to **lock lips with Parisian passion,** treasure the pleasure of this unique and sexy way to simultaneously **take her into your mouth and your heart.**

Très bien!

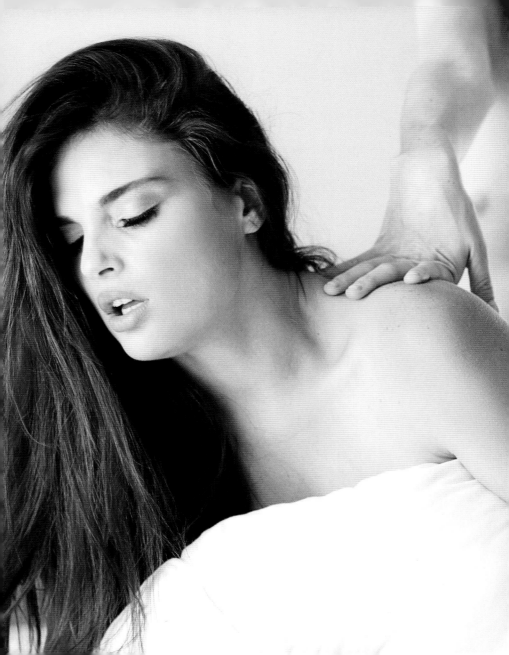

85 All About You

Love has nothing to do with what you are expecting to get, only what you are expecting to give, which is everything.
—Katharine Hepburn

Altruism is a natural human inclination, and for some, a rather powerful urge. Enormous satisfaction comes from gratifying another, especially a lover. **Pleasing you pleases her.**

Pleasure is her right and yours. Know how to receive pleasure so that in turn, you can give it. Selflessly surrender to every whim of her mouth, hands, body, and words as she meets your needs and indulges your desires.

As dreamy as you become while under her tender loving care, endeavor to pay attention as she directs this play that's (seemingly) all about you. Her actions hint at what she'd like done to her when it's your turn to bestow pleasure.

Your desire elicits hers. Turning you on and getting you off is a turn-on for *her*. Your arousal arouses her. Your wetness makes her wet.

Hearing your **soulful sighs** as the pleasure she's providing consumes you will make her want to keep on **blissing you out** all night long! Your faint moan is **the sexiest music to her ears.**

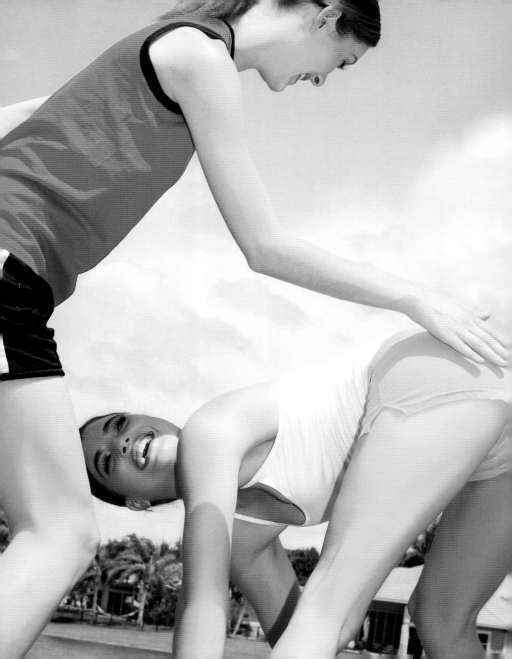

86 Team Player

Pass, set, crush!

Love is not for the passive. Passion is reserved for the dynamic. **Be participants,** and together, join a team.

As they say in beach volleyball, *all it takes is a little sand and some balls.*

Find out how strong you both are, and how weak—**the size of her fight and the size of your heart.** Healthy competition not only builds character, it reveals it.

Fueled by the heat of the day and the fresh sea air, you and she release *the self* in pursuit of a higher purpose. It's a thrill to be a crucial cog in a fierce, dedicated, hardworking machine, contributing your ambition, enthusiasm, and prowess toward a shared goal.

Nothing worthwhile comes easy. And winning never gets old. **Dig deep,** mentally and physically. Put in your all, and then give a little more.

Doing what's best for your bodies will also boost performance in your one-on-one bedroom bouts.

Bump it to her, set it to her, one more time!

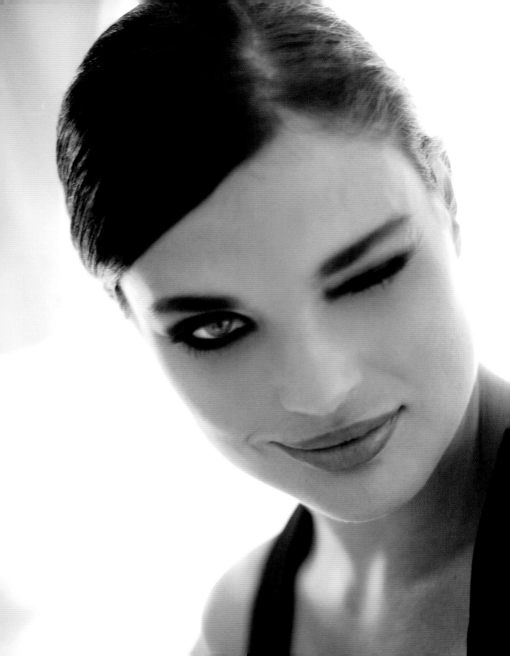

87 Mischief

What are friends for if you can't exploit them for your own amusement?

Utilize a private lexicon when you and she are in public.

Language is sexy. Allusions are intriguing.

Shared wordplay endows lovers with **the thrill of willful rebelliousness,** the intimacy of a secret, and the self-satisfaction gained through cleverness.

Everyone is confident in some situations and shy in others. Counter social anxieties as you and your accomplice control the scene, seeking new ways to let loose these double entendres of your own creation.

Mischievously greet a clueless pal ...

Hey! How's the daily grind treating you?

... while catching her twinkling eye to acknowledge what you're actually announcing **between the lines.**

Right now, I'm picturing you on top of me, perfectly crushing me with your lovely breasts as you rub yourself hard.

Secret message received!

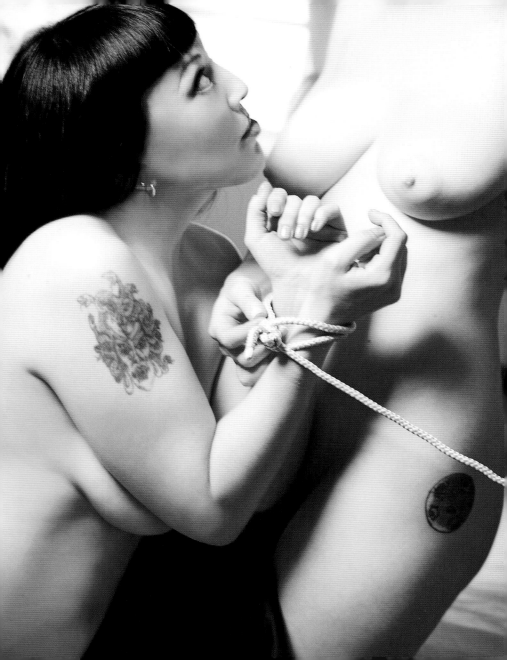

88 All Wrapped Up

Provocative games inspire fantasies and break the ice for discovering and sharing proclivities.

Knottily wrap her bare or nearly nude body from head to toe with silk fabric and ribbons or rope.

Once she's adorned in her fashionable trusses, take a lingering moment to admire your intricate design as her senses absorb and react to the inventive experience. Then unwrap her like the stylish present she is, gradually releasing her from her binding predicament. When finally free, she'll likely be game for a frisky round of hand-to-hand combat.

Wrap yourself for her.

Wrap yourselves tightly together using cellophane or resistance bands, and then explore and invent ways to twist, turn, thrust, and rub in sync.

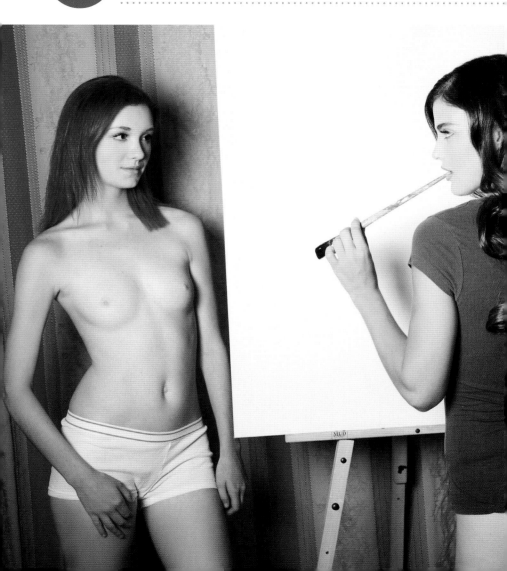

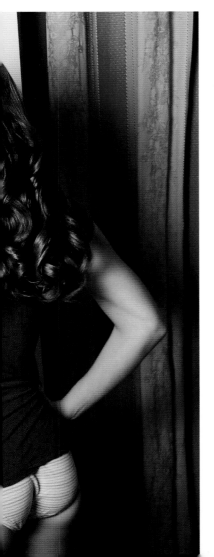

Like sex, the arts offer an opportunity to connect outside the encapsulated self.

Too much time is spent processing information, and too little actually thinking and feeling—especially deeply and sensually. The brain's habits often belie the promise that lies within. Art, science, and philosophy elevate you, moving you both beyond patterns of everyday thinking into the sublime.

Provoke her instincts and **churn her creative juices.** Wander galleries for treasures old and new. As your creative energies commune, challenge preconceived notions of beauty and influence. **Celebrate your illuminations.**

Through art's unifying power, you and she make the nuanced connections that will inspire you both to grow and go further.

Your *ponds* are bigger and deeper than you think.

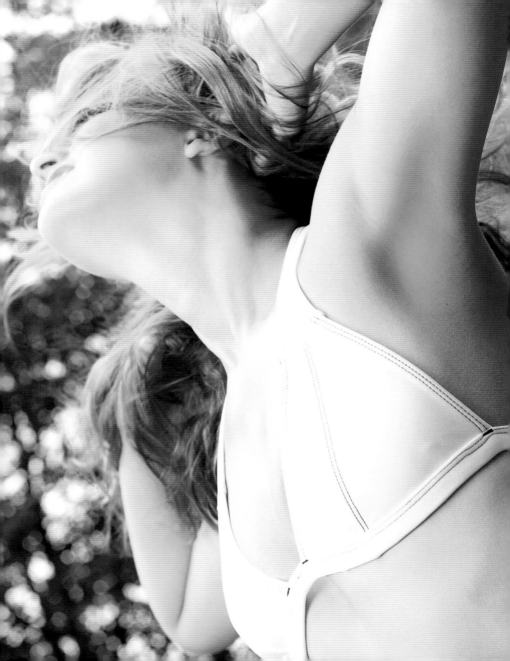

90 Lose Your Senses

She needs *you* to need *her*.

She wants you to be irrational over her—to lose your senses, deliriously infatuated and consumed with longing.

Once you lose hold of your heart, the head follows. Her ability to completely shift your brain from reason to intuition pleases her.

Toss your common sense to the wind.

To be sure, she favors a calm, cool, and reliable partner when the daily push comes to shove. Yet **she'll always long to drive you wild** and ignite your unbridled passion.

Be impetuous.

Curbing your emotions—especially spontaneous and amorous ones— is an overrated attribute of so-called maturity.

Love her truly, madly, and deeply.

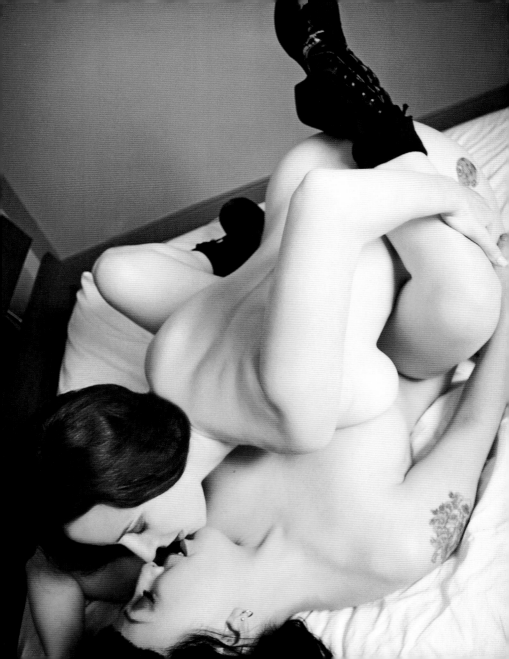

91 Keep Those Shoes On

Objects, ideas, and certain parts of the body can elicit a reverence known as a fetish. The more obsessive, in fact, can't be sexually gratified without the presence of the fixation. For others, whose attachment to a particular object of desire is mere affection, **fetish play** can be a real kick!

Whether you spend your days in business suits or sweatsuits, a sexy dress code in the bedroom should be unyieldingly enforced. Exactly how this style is to be characterized, night to night, is much less strict. When a woman is working her style and feeling good, **it's her attitude that seduces.**

Footwear strikes a chord on many levels. Some shoes are designed for seduction, while the shape and texture of others will convey authority or speed. Whether you surprise her with stiletto heels, *bad-ass* boots, or personalized sneakers, the visual stimulation is immediate. She's **smitten with her nonconforming kitten.**

The scenario creates an arousing urgency, implying that in the throes of passion, there's simply no time or opportunity to remove them.

Ultimately, the sexiest thing about wearing your shoes to bed, beyond the thrill of *knockin' boots* while knocking boots, is the manner in which she gets you out of them!

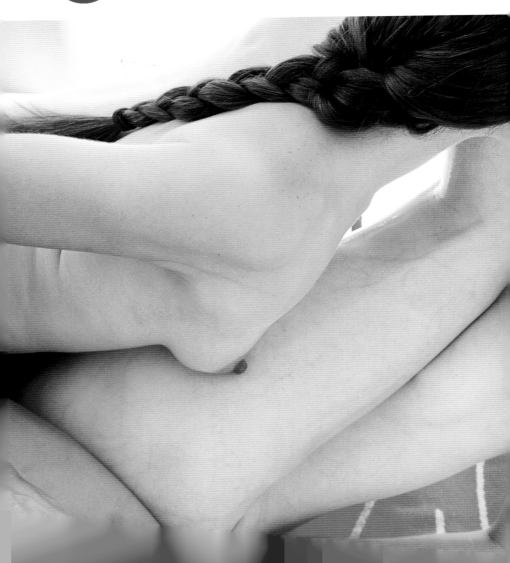

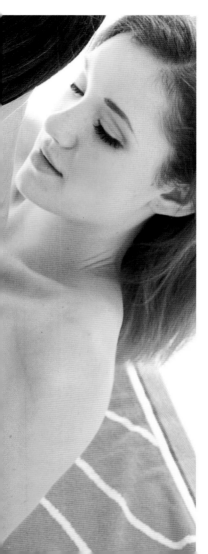

Employ two of your most beautiful assets to anoint her body with a melting sensuality.

When combined with the natural wetness of your arousal, massage oil as a sensual medium creates a distinctive alchemy for a purely surface-oriented sexual encounter.

This **slow and sexy spreading** of oil surpasses typical skin-to-skin contact— with inunction, you give her an entirely new sensorial experience. *What sweetness!*

Cup a breast to direct the painterly path of your nipple across her provocative hills and kissable valleys.

Her skin is on high alert. Your explicit trail of oil excites her skin and her mind way beyond the soothing, broad strokes of massage.

Make her **drip with sultry eros.**

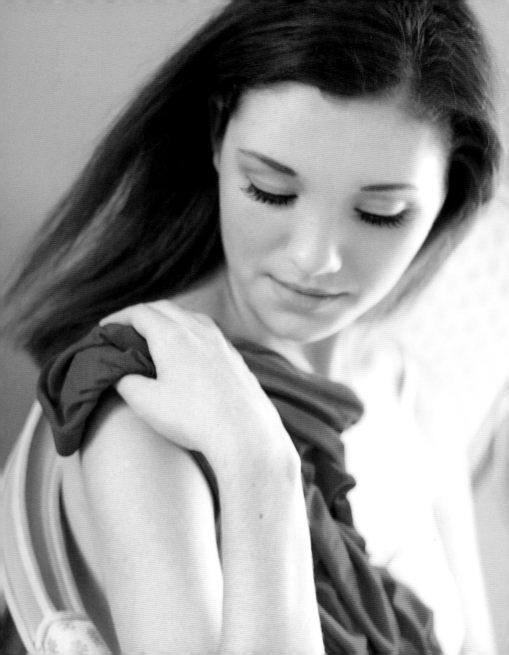

93 Petite Madeleine

She came to me again in a scent.

Few impressions are as potent as sensory memory. Of the senses, the olfactory is the most intoxicating. The brain immediately attaches an emotion to a smell, and can retain the emotion long after the stimulus fades away.

For the author Proust, a whiff and then a taste of a small cake extraordinarily returned him to his childhood, to a time when he was happy, loving, and being loved.

Infuse yourself beneath the surface of her consciousness.

When lovers intertwine, their **chemistries mingle** and react. The scent of arousal has staying power.

I woke up to her next to me, closed my eyes again, and inhaled the fragrance of her hair. I wanted to touch her but held back— I didn't want to wake her. I drew in her scent again, a deep breath, and then rolled onto my back. Last night's amazing sex raced through my head and I reached down to feel myself. I want to do it all again. Have her do it all again to me. I pressed my naked body into her soft, warm back and kissed her out of her slumber . . .

Set off a pang in her heart. When you're not with her, she'll ache to return even fleetingly to that moment when you so exquisitely and sensorially invaded her.

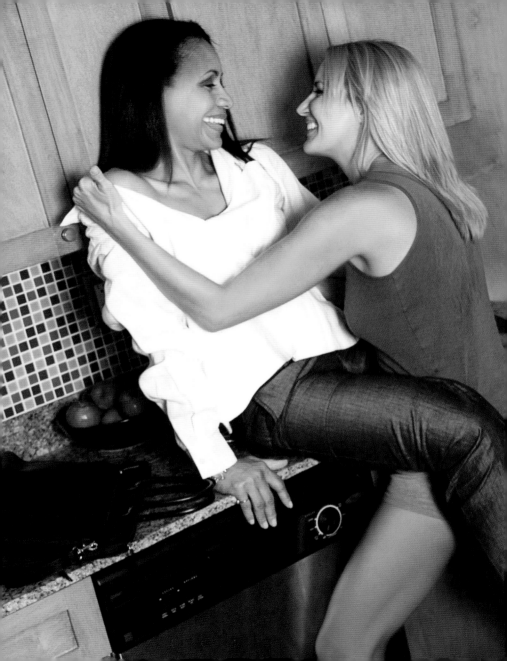

94 Crack of Dawn

It's time for *her privates* to *rise and shine.*

Fool around at the break of day. She's likely most open to new impressions and sensations in the morning.

Breakfast nookie can be assertive or gentle, and certainly isn't limited to any particular room. Suspend her daybreak ritual with a seductive invitation left atop freshly laid-out towels that reads:

> *What happens in the kitchen stays in the kitchen.*
> *Meet there in 5!*

Work up an appetite with some **heavy petting in the pantry.** Spank her bottom *over easy* with her favorite spatula as she braces herself against a shelf of canned goods.

Send her to work with a smile on her face. Slip into her car as she's about to depart, and then *suck her hen* while she squirms with delight in the driver's seat.

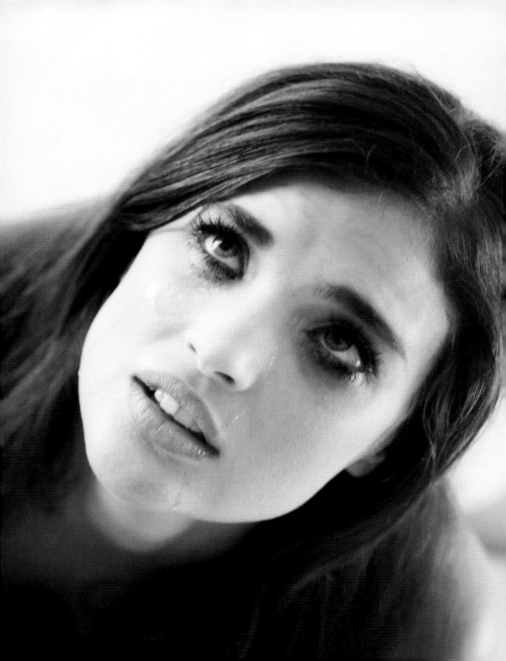

95 Heart on Sleeve

Dare to be transparent in an increasingly anonymous world.

Great love and great achievements call for great risk.

Maintaining an air of intrigue doesn't mean being so reserved and elusive that she becomes concerned about your consistency and trustworthiness.

Openly display your emotions. Reveal hopes, dreams, worries, and experiences. Bare your soul and expose yourself to her gaze and scrutiny. If she stays, it'll be for *you*, scars and all.

A fierce and willful woman is seductive, yet a constant show of courage won't place a stronghold on her heart. Allow her to know a trace of your weakness. Disclosure fortifies a relationship.

Vulnerability captivates. It's real and it's raw.

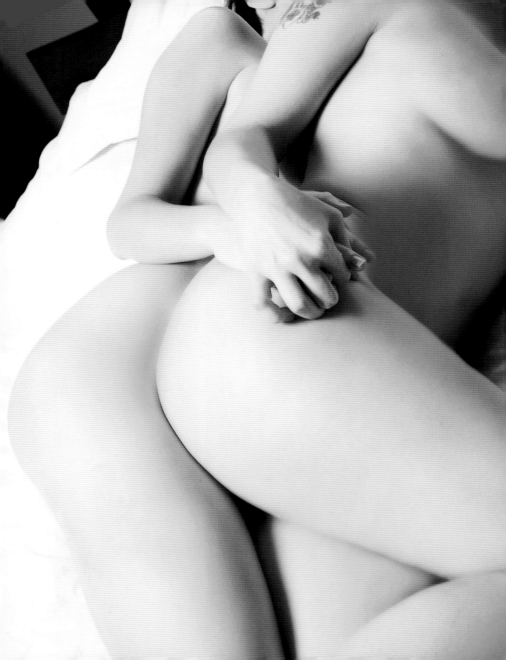

96 Hold

Biology takes over when love happens.

Women are hormonally complicated. The effects on her body and brain vary greatly, and—especially with regard to sexual response—are highly dependent on levels and interaction. When oxytocin interacts with estrogen, for example, that's when her connection to you is its most intense.

Your touch, anywhere on her body, escalates her desire to be touched further. Sexual attraction and love are emotional reactions fashioned in the brain and susceptible to conditioning. Thus, once you and she are enjoying each other fully, the mere sight of you can **elevate her hormone levels;** hearing your voice can release within her a wave of oxytocin. Your touch—although essential sexually, socially, and psychologically to nurture and fulfill her—is no longer essential for her to desire you.

When flowing through her pleasure-ridden body, this enterprising hormone can make for a more powerful orgasm. And upon climaxing, another burst of oxytocin surges into her bloodstream, boosting her desire to cuddle, nuzzle, and spoon with you as **she basks in the soothing afterglow of scrumptious sex.**

What more can one be sure of than that which one holds in one's arms, at the moment one holds it in one's arms.
    —Colette

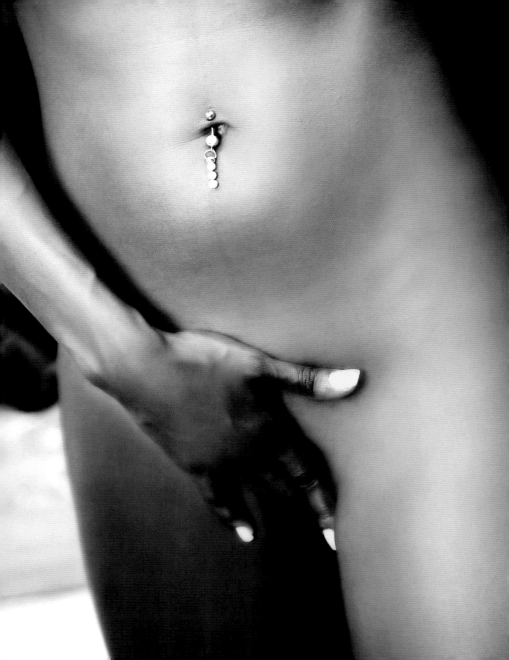

97 Bliss at Your Fingertips

When a woman enters another woman, it's most often her fingers that first cross the threshold to feel the wet warmth inside.

Palm her *mountain of Venus* and with your lightly lubricated fingers, feel the folds of her vulva's outer and inner lips. Trace around her vaginal vestibule.

Experiment with different types of touch: a rhythmic stroke, the tickle of a two-fingered strum, and the startling titillation of a light pluck.

Lovingly caress the sides of her clitoris, place your fingertips on her clitoral hood, and *rub her round and round.*

Use her natural vaginal fluid, and add lube, if desired, to **moisten the margins of her entrance.** Slip a finger inside. Additional fingers can join in as the angle of action allows, as is desired by both lovers, and as she expands to welcome you.

Continue to move in and out of her while your thumb meets and greets her clit's aroused, emerging head with each penetrative plunge. Your free hand can take over for more controlled clitoral stimulation, or wander.

Treasure the privilege of being inside a woman. Stay inside her while you bring her to climax. Give new meaning to the phrase, *You've got her wrapped around your finger.*

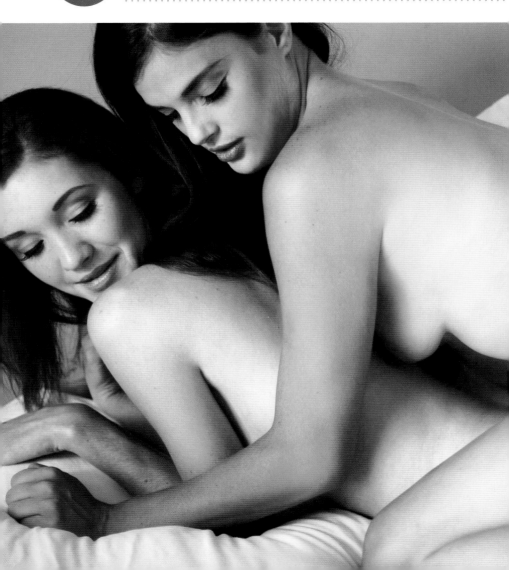

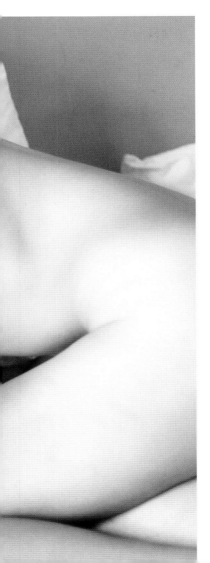

Land on planet Pleasure's most heavenly moon.

Sex requires friction and excitement to fully inspire both the body and the mind. **She'll be mad about the moment when she first feels your wetness.**

After a few playful bounces and pussy presses, lay prone on her, pressing your breasts into her back, perhaps gripping a shoulder for added leverage. **Rub on her sweet cheeks** until one of you steers the encounter in a new direction, or if so moved, until you climax atop her lovely ass.

Sometimes this type of *sexcapade* begins as an innocent back massage. The oil you lovingly spread across her hot buns provides an extra slippery slope to slide around on.

After your *backside ride* culminates in a rippling climax, reach between her legs, as she's certain to be excited, aroused by **feeling you undulating all over her.**

It's her turn to straddle your ass and *ride your landscape.*

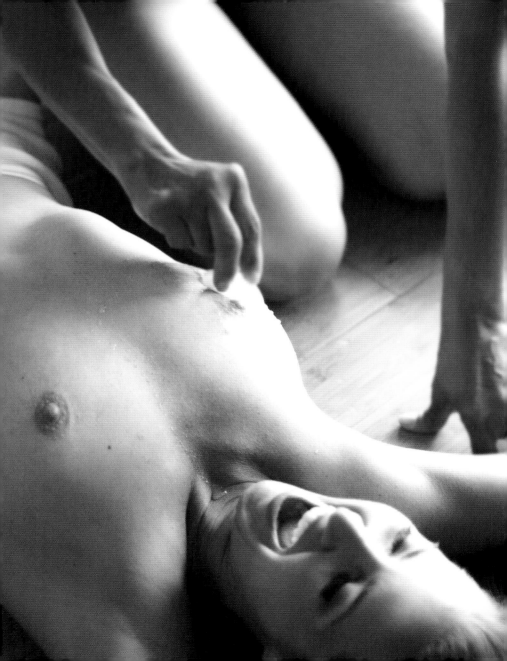

99 Is It Warm in Here?

Alter her temperature.

Temperature play is a topping technique that requires an atmosphere of safety for her nerves to shift into low and relax, despite her aroused body. In this state, her body has a higher tolerance, so changes in temperature provide vigorous sensations.

Briefly twirl an ice cube on and around her nipples. Glide it, melting, down her neck and along her body. Follow each sweep with a puff of your warm breath.

With ice chips or a cube in your mouth, bury your face in her warm pussy and **give her clit a start with your numbed tongue.**

Just when her body and mind believe they can predict what's coming, **crank up the heat.** Light a body candle and ask permission. If she says yes, blow out the candle and tilt it so that wax drips onto her delicate skin. Keep in mind that the closer you are, the hotter it'll be. Neophytes may dip fingertips into the liquid wax and then touch. Target a less sensitive (and hairless) area such as her lower back or the palm of her hand. **Her arousal increases her receptiveness.**

This feverish fun is about progression, amplified rushes of energy, and colliding responses. Trace with an ice cube the area onto which you just dripped wax to superbly surprise her nerve endings and mystify her senses.

The agony and the ecstasy.

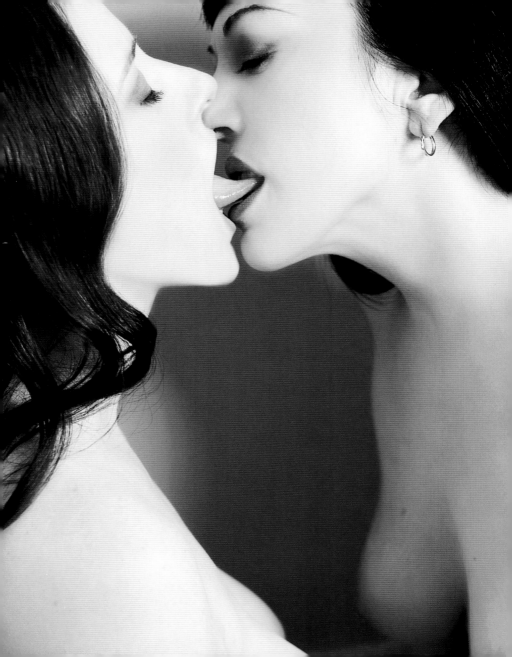

100 Bite Your Tongue

Don't wake the neighbors. Don't shout it from the rooftops. **Don't speak.** For an entire session of lovemaking, including foreplay, don't say a single word.

Silence is extraordinarily powerful and intriguingly sexy.

Hushed lovers connect when compelled to express their feelings, wishes, intentions, and pleasure more inventively.

Everyone appreciates acknowledgment, especially in the bedroom. During your next sexual skirmish, communicate your desire and delight through only the tempo and vigor of your movements.

Lick your lips and take a deep breath as shes glances up from between your legs. Clasp her hand or grip her body when you're nearing climax.

While fingering her, take her fingers and insert them too, mingling them with yours as they move in and out of her.

This hot move, accompanied by your deliberate gaze and smile, silently communicates volumes.

Inside you, I feel real.

101 Verve

She's as wet as October, and so, so delicious. You feel you could spend your life between her legs.

Gild her lily after you've brought her to climax with the vivacious attentions of your mouth—encircle her silken labia with a slow, loving lick.

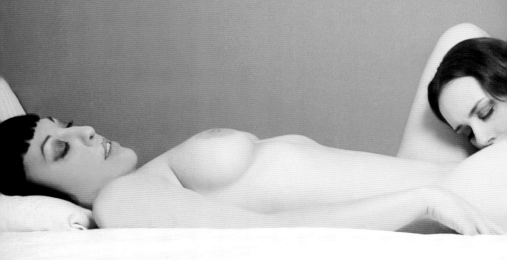

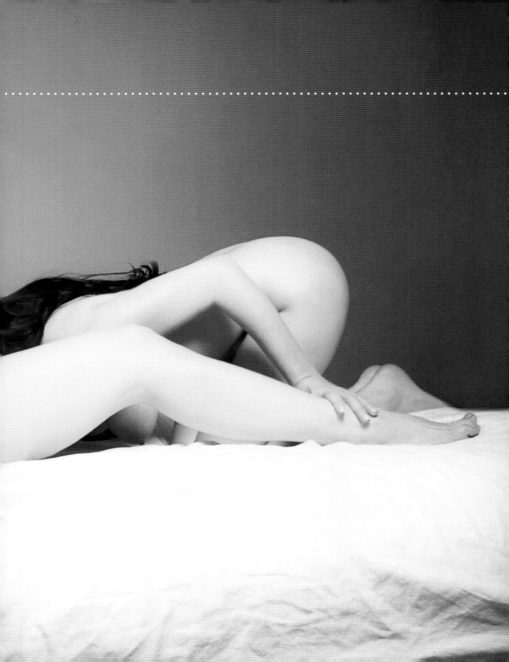

LEXICON

Sweet spots are tangible and intangible places on or within a woman's body, mind, heart, and soul, that when touched in a way that she enjoys, give her great satisfaction, fulfillment, and pleasure.

Climax is often interchanged with the term orgasm. Descriptive phrases include *orgasmic peak, zenith, happy ending, untangle her tingle, plateau, crescendo,* and *launch her rocket.*

Wetness refers to the moisture she emits via her vaginal walls upon her arousal, as in, *"she's getting so wet"* and *"taste her sweet sugar."* The fluid is also called her *juices, fresh dew, tea,* and *natural emission of passion.*

To *gild her lily* is to resolutely lick her labia just after she climaxes.

When two women have sex, it may be referred to as *knockin' boots, a game of flats, getting busy, the in and out, making love, tribadism or tribbing* (non-penetrative sex during which a woman rubs her pussy against her lover for stimulation), *fucking,* and the *bump and grind.*

Breasts are sometimes called *tits, titties, tatas,* and *her girls.*

Mountain of Venus (mons veneris) is the soft, external mound over her pelvic bone.

Genitals are often called *nether regions, naughty bits,* and *privates.*

Labia are her genitals' inner (minora) and outer (majora) lips, also known as her *lower lips, labiacious petals,* and *velvet folds.*

Her *pussy* is her lower genitals, encompassing the internal bits as well as the external (vulva). Her *pussy* may be affectionately referred to as *her bizness, la la, hoo ha, little duchess, petite praline, muff, flower, cunt, lower lady love, honey pot, cookie jar, velvet forest, vajajay, trim, pie, priscilla's punchbowl, pudding, honey jar, her ocean,* and *fur-lined teacup.*

A *pompoir* is likened to a genital hug, occurring when a woman flexes and squeezes her vaginal muscles, gripping the inserted sex toy or fingers.

Her clitoris is also called her *clit, princess in a boat, pleasure center* (not to be confused with the pleasure center or reward circuit located within the brain), *pleasure hub* or *nub, little papaya, bud,* and *lotus stem of love.*

Her G-spot is sometimes called her *pleasure sponge, magic spot,* and *her clit's back door.*

Specific areas of her anal region may be affectionately referred to as her *tail zone, buttocks, ass, sweet cheeks, derrière, biscuit buns, puckering starfish* (rectum), *P-spot* (perineum), *heavenly moon, hot fanny cakes,* and her *booty.*

Jilling, jillin', and *jilling off,* refer to masturbation or the art of sexual self-pleasuring. *Mutual jillin'* is when women simultaneously perform this on each other.

Cunnilingus is the act of performing oral sex on a woman. This lovemaking technique is also affectionately known as *sipping her tea, going downtown, polishing her jewels, muff-diving, sipping her rose, sucking her hen* (the *hen* referring specifically to her clitoris), and *lip service.*

A *double header,* also known as a *garden party* or a *dutch tulip* (depending on the positions of the lovers' bodies), is the sexual act of two women simultaneously performing oral sex on one other.

Stud muffin' is when a woman performs oral sex on another woman who's wearing a sex toy strap-on kit.

When she dons a strap-on sex toy kit, the harnessed dildo is known as her *clit extension* or *her member.*

Sexual activity among three women is known as a *treble play, ménage a trois,* and *threefold.*

Vanilla conventionally refers to the missionary position, yet also defines routine, most often, a couple's routine with regard to their lovemaking.

Splosh or *sploshing* is sexy food play.

To pack or *be packing* is to place either a specially-designed package such as a dildo, or one of ingenuity such as a balled up pair of socks, underneath her clothing atop her clitoris to augment her clit's presence.

Rimming is oral sex performed on her anal region, also referred to as *tongue and groove*. To *rim bareback* is to do it with no safe sex barrier between the mouth and the anus.

Rubber johnnies are condoms. A *dental dam* is a sheath (usually made from rubber or latex) used during oral sex to prevent the spreading of infection and sexually transmitted diseases (STDs).

SAFETY NOTES

This book's intention is to inspire and entertain. The ideas and techniques described are for the utilization of informed, consenting adults with common sense and sound judgment, and in no way represent the full knowledge required for safely and legally undertaking them.

Safe, sane, and consensual is the standard to uphold without exception during intimate encounters. When pleasing her sweet spot, improvisation and the power of surprise are, by and large, applauded. However, prior to and throughout engaging in any sexual act, especially when it involves an element of risk or danger, the plan must be clearly communicated and consensually agreed upon. Make use of a safe word that when engaged, signals and stops the action.

Keep yourself, your environment, and all accessories clean. Choose and properly use quality sensual products and accessories that are designed for a particular activity. Follow all use, cleaning and disinfecting, and care instructions.

For anal, vaginal, food, and all other play, take care to prevent the transfer of bacteria or the initiation or spreading of infection. Discard and apply new condoms, dental dams, and related safe sex accessories, and maintain cleanliness throughout every encounter, especially when a sex toy travels from hand to mouth to nether regions. Choose and plentifully use a good lube. Avoid glycerin, found in many water-based lubes, as sugar can lead to infections. Glycerin-free, silicone-based lubes tend to be free of harmful chemicals and stay slippery longer.

If your lover or target of seduction is pregnant, many of the sensory "rules" fall to the wayside, often due to hormonal variations. Foods, drinks, herbs, lotions, oils, and other sensual accessories often act and interact in unexpected ways. Safeguard against allergic reactions and other adverse effects through education and the consultation of qualified experts.

ACKNOWLEDGMENTS

Everything is better when you do it with someone special. I'm grateful to the many exceptional individuals who shared in bringing *Her Sweet Spot* to life. Aaron Wehner saw promise in an idea and wholeheartedly gave the green light to explore and realize this book. My spot-on editor, Sara Golski, with patience and enthusiasm, focused my tangential thoughts so that the book's gifted designer, Colleen Cain, could shape our vision. Many thanks to everyone at Ten Speed Press who contributed in their own way to this project's success.

Special thanks to photographer extraordinaire, the *terribly girly* Janette Valentine, and her team of fierce women, Gail Greiner, Dr. Al Damus, Berta, Bonnie, and Bob, Allison and Michael Macleod, Deborah Lile, Judith Ellen Krout, Mike Osborn, Karen Prince, Sean Moore and his right hand, Meredith, Kitty Burrows, Mamie's Catering, Nikki and Nate, Edna Lavinia & Associates, all the beautiful people who in various ways and times throughout my life were behind my pen or in front of my lens, and to my talented, devoted, and passionate family, Aimée, and our Tweedster of Love.

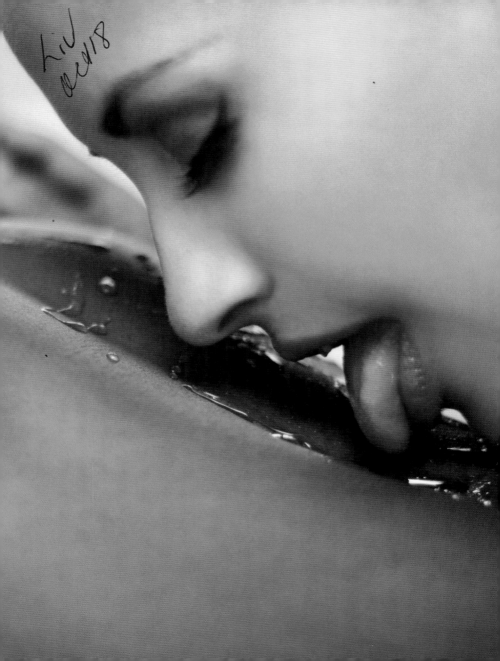